DEMENTIA AND DRIVING

When A Person Living With Dementia Needs To Stop Driving

Debra Ricker, OTR/L, CDT, DRS

Contents

About The Author- Debbie Ricker 5

Introduction 7

Ch. 1 What changes with normal aging 13

Ch. 2 Reasons older adults give up driving 23

Ch. 3 Health professional & family's role 31

Ch. 4 Not normal aging: Its effects 39

Ch. 5 Mild cognitive impairment 47

Ch. 6 Dementia 51

Ch. 7 Alzheimer's Disease 55

Ch. 8 Lewy Body Dementia 59

Ch. 9 Frontotemporal Dementia 63

Ch. 10 Vascular Dementia 67

Ch. 11 How cognitive abilities are assessed 69

Ch. 12 Driving is a priviledge, not a 79

Ch. 13 How dementia affects driving and reasoning 91

Ch. 14 Research on driving and Dementia 97

Ch. 15 Is your loved one save to drive? 103

Ch. 16 Legal consequeces of driving with dementia...........113

Ch. 17 Case studies...115

Ch. 18 Statistics & research...135

Ch. 19 Alternative transportations.......................................143

Ch. 20 In conclusion...147

Bibliography...151

About The Author

Debbie Ricker, OTR/L, DRS, CDT

Debbie Ricker graduated from Loma Linda University with a bachelor's degree in Occupational Therapy. She spent the first twenty years of her career working in various psychiatric settings-state hospitals, adult day healthcare, gero-psych units, and short-term psychiatric hospitals. Ms. Ricker founded a business creating therapy programs for psychiatric patients, including occupational therapy, recreation therapy, music therapy, and art therapy. She went on to specialize in working with older adults including those living with dementia and is currently a Certified Dementia Trainer. Ricker became a Driving Rehabilitation Specialist, founded The Adaptive Driving Center in 2001, and specialized in driving assessments for older adults. Most of her clients have been diagnosed with some type of cognitive impairment. Other diagnoses she assists with include Parkinson's disease, stroke, and brain tumors.

Introduction

I wrote this book to meet the need for more information on how dementia causes impaired driving, to highlight the shortage of driving assessors who are experts in the field, to address the lack of awareness in the medical community, and finally, to point out the tsunami of older adults who are being diagnosed with dementia and are still driving, and how this affects road safety for everyone. You are an integral part of spreading the word about the dangers of driving with dementia, as well as how to address the problem.

While all forms of dementia affect driving ability, we will often refer to Alzheimer's disease since it is the most common form of dementia. According to the Alzheimer's Association, someone in the United States develops dementia every 66 seconds. 100% of these individuals will be unsafe to drive at some point in the progression of their disease. Unsafe drivers need to stop driving BEFORE they harm others or themselves-- or before they get lost and suffer the negative consequences. There are many people who are driving with dementia, not only putting them at risk but putting all those around them at risk, and the driver with dementia is at high risk for getting lost. Example 1: a gentleman drove and was lost for nine hours before finally being stopped by a police officer, who gave him the assistance he needed to get home. His license was taken away on the spot and his car was impounded. Imagine the terror and frustration this man felt! Part of the dementia process is losing the ability to make good decisions, solve problems, or even have the awareness of needing help. Example 2: a woman stated that she got lost, and the clue that helped her realize she was really lost- all the signs were in Spanish. She knew that she was no longer in California by looking at the signs. She didn't realize on the four-hour drive to Mexico that she was lost. But both were driving- and they had been driving for hours while they were too incapacitated to drive safely at all. Example 3: A representative from a California state senator's office called and stated that the senator wanted a constituent to be "tested and passed, and get his license back", and urged for a driving assessment as "quickly as possible". When I arrived at the individual's home, he stated, "That officer was ageist! He took my license away on the spot! There was no sign stating, 'no left turn' and I made a left turn. He stopped me and he took my license away and impounded my car! He was totally out of line taking my car and my license. I just want to drive, and I want you to help me get my license back! I have a picture to prove that I was okay to turn left!" He immediately went to retrieve the picture and showed it to me. The sign in the picture said, "Right turn only". Obviously, the officer at the scene was so concerned about his driving, and probably during the interaction with the driver, that he decided to impound the car and take the driver's license on the spot. This driver did not pass the driving assessment with me and was advised to stop driving. He was very upset at the recommendation to stop driving, but there were obvious errors during the written portion of the test, as well as the driving portion of the test, that indicated he was no longer safe to drive.

The complications of driving while under the influence of Mild Cognitive Impairment or dementia are not common knowledge. Many family members are either naïve about their loved one continuing to drive after being diagnosed with any degree of cognitive impairment, or they turn a blind eye to the problem because they don't want the burden of being responsible for driving their loved one to all the destinations that are part of daily living when they can no longer drive themselves. One question that we ask these reluctant family members is, would you allow your children to ride with your parent/grandparent/aunt/uncle?" Often the family members will answer "no", yet they allow their loved one to continue driving. If the loved one is not safe to drive with family members in the car, they are probably no longer safe to drive at all.

So, the problem is two-fold: one is the issue of evaluating whether the person's cognitive impairment renders them unsafe to drive; the other is the necessity of the family members or healthcare providers to face this major issue head on and then deal with it. These issues affect the safety not only of the person who is impaired, but countless others who may have random interactions with that driver.

This book gives you the information you need to confront this very difficult issue to the benefit of both you and your loved one. It is not an easy issue to deal with, but it is truly important that you deal with it. It can be a matter of life and death, at its most extreme. It is a matter of everyday peace of mind for you, safety for your loved one and all those others out there that your loved one happens to interact with while driving.

This book will give you the foundation of the most common types of dementia, including how the brain is affected and the symptoms that are common with each diagnosis. You are welcome to read the book chapter by chapter, or simply use the information that is relevant to you. The chapters are listed by subject matter so you can quickly turn to the chapters that are most relevant to what you are researching.

Chapter 1

What Changes with Normal Aging

True or False: Most older adults cease or restrict their

own driving when they experience changes in their ability

to drive.

If you answered "true", you are correct. Our senses typically change as we age- these senses include vision, hearing, taste, touch, and smell. With vision, light and images are processed through the eyes, the images are interpreted in the brain, and then we typically respond to the images with movement. When driving we must process those images quickly. The pupils control how much light is processed before reaching the brain. At age 60 your pupils can decrease to 1/3 the size that your pupils were at age 20. You will probably have more difficulty with glare recovery after passing a car at night with the headlights on- especially if the car has halogen headlights. It is common to have reduced peripheral vision with aging. Some people develop floaters in the eyes, which can be distracting when driving.

Most older adults do restrict their own driving when they experience more challenges when driving. But that entails still having the awareness that changes are occurring. The population that are usually reluctant to restrict their driving are the individuals who are living with dementia. They have lost their ability to observe whether they can drive safely and will not typically see that their driving skills are so impaired that they can no longer drive safely.

With age, the ability to focus on small objects/print is compromised- ever see someone in a restaurant, putting on glasses and taking them off, moving the menu closer and farther away? They are attempting to adjust for changing vision. The ability to switch from near to far becomes diminished, and during driving includes being able to look at the gauges in the car to determine if we have gas in the tank, or what speed we are going, and then look up to observe the traffic flow and make adjustments as needed. We need to have good peripheral vision so that we can spot motorcycles/vehicles/cyclists driving up beside our vehicle or a car that is attempting to change lanes near us. Our pupils must react quickly to light changes as we drive from a tree lined, shady street to a sunny area. This process slows as we age.

Most people develop arthritis as they age, which can impair a driver's ability to steer accurately, as well as handle all the controls in the vehicle. It is also common for aging drivers to have back and neck pain, which can certainly complicate driving, and make it difficult to look over the shoulder prior to making lane changes. An individual can have changes in hearing, or loss of high frequency sounds. We experienced this in one driving assessment when the driver attempted to turn in front of two emergency vehicles with lights and sirens on.

The human brain was not created to multitask, but driving requires ultimate shifts in attention- being able to remember state driving laws, to read all the gauges and symbols in the car, remember the meaning of all the street signs and signal lights, attend to all the vehicles and pedestrians around a car, and plan ahead for changing traffic patterns. The brain has slower processing skills as we age, and it takes an older adult a longer time to process all the information taken in through the eyes. The aging brain needs more time and information to decide how to respond to each situation. Sensory perception may become weaker, and may be very impaired, as in the example of individuals with neuropathy in the hands or feet.

How does vision change as we age normally? Dynamic visual acuity is the ability to see and process information about a moving object. That means that our eyes and brain need to be able to see and process moving cars, trucks, bicycles, motorcycles, animals, pedestrians- anything that might be on or near the road. We need to have good depth perception- we need to know how far away we are from vehicles and pedestrians, parked cars, and any other objects nearby. All these changes in vision are magnified in the person living with dementia. The most common accident that an individual living with dementia will cause is turning left in front of oncoming traffic. This is because they lose depth perception early in the dementia process, which causes them to lose the ability to see how far away (or close) the vehicles are, or how fast they are approaching.

In occupational therapy terms, we use the term **useful field of view**. It is the area that you can see **and** cognitively process so that you can interpret which reactions you need to perform when driving.

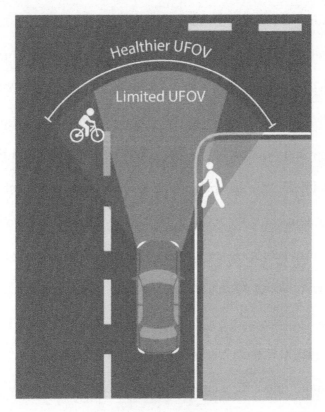

Illustration Meaning:

A driver with a normal useful field of view will be able to see and process this entire scene. That means they will see the cyclist and the pedestrian and will plan on stopping to allow these individuals to cross the street. A driver with cognitive impairment and impaired useful field of view will only see the lighter area, are unable to see and plan for the cyclist and pedestrian crossing in front and are likely to cause an accident because they can't plan ahead.

Demonstration: These three scenarios will help you further understand how cognitive impairment and dementia will impair vision and ability to interpret what an individual is able to see and then respond to in their environment. The first activity demonstrates mild cognitive impairment or the beginning stages of dementia and their visual field. The second activity demonstrates middle stages of dementia and what these individuals can see and process. The third activity demonstrates visual field for an individual in last stages of dementia.

Activity 1: make a "scuba mask" with your hands: Curl your left hand into a 'C' shape and place it around your eye. The back of your hand will be the outside of the "mask". Now do the same with your other hand and connect thumb to thumb over the bridge of your nose, and your fingertips of both hands at your brow line. As if you are shielding your eyes from the sun. In beginning stages of dementia, that is the area that an individual can see and process. In middles stages of dementia, it is like looking through binoculars.

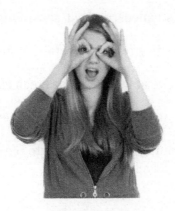

Activity 2: make a pair of "binoculars" by curling your fingers to your thumbs and put your binoculars in front of your eyes. Similar to the figure above but mimicking the shape of binoculars. Imagine trying to drive with such limited peripheral vision!

In the end stages of dementia, it is as if you have monocular vision- you can only see out of one eye.

Activity 3: to visualize this, make a "binocular" over one eye, keeping the other eye closed. Try to imagine how you would drive with such limited vision. You can see how, based on visual changes alone, driving becomes very impaired as dementia progresses. And useful field of view is only one aspect of driving.

We also need to have the ability to see similarly colored objects, which is called contrast sensitivity. If there is a green car driving in front of a section of green bushes and trees, we need to be able to see that green car in front of the greenery. Or if it is a foggy day, and there is a gray car driving near us, our eyes must be able to see the contrast and differentiate between the two.

We also need perceptual reaction time, which is the ability to see objects and quickly respond to what we are seeing. Glare recovery is the ability to recover from oncoming headlights. Have you ever seen opposing traffic at night, with halogen headlights? It can take a while for our eyes to adjust once the oncoming traffic passes, and as we age that process slows down.

As mentioned earlier, we need good peripheral vision so that we can see what is happening at the edges of the windshield, and to the sides of the vehicle. We especially need to be aware of smaller cars, cyclists, pedestrians, animals-anything that may impede our safety or a human's or animal's safety.

Finally, the last type of vision that changes with normal aging is light/dark adaptation, such as entering and exiting a tunnel. If we are driving in bright sun and then enter a tunnel or darkened area, it typically takes 20 to 30 minutes for the eyes to fully adjust to the darkness. Night vision will become more impaired as we age due to decreased light passing through the eyes and can cause blurry or impaired vision when facing the glare of headlights and streetlights.

Driving is typically viewed as a "right" and not a privilege. Remember when you first got your driver's license? It was a symbol that you were now responsible enough to drive a car, to go anywhere you wanted to go, and not have to rely on your parents to drive you. It is also a symbol of becoming an adult, of having freedom and independence. The ability to go where you want to go, when you want to go. But the truth is that driving is not a right- it is a privilege. Whether we are 16 or 56 or 86, we need to prove, every time that we drive, that we are still capable of driving safely.

The changes outlined in this chapter- normal changes that may occur as we grow older- can threaten that privilege of driving. Since being able to drive is a major factor in being able to be independent, our awareness of the changes may be compromised by the loss of independence they entail, even for those of us without dementia. It can't be emphasized enough- every driver with a diagnosis of dementia will reach a point where they are no longer safe to drive.

What is the most common accident that a driver with dementia causes? A left-hand turn with oncoming traffic, because dementia robs a person of depth perception, so the driver is unable to determine how far away the traffic is or how fast the cars are approaching.

Chapter 2

Reasons Older Adults Give Up Driving

As noted, it is common for individuals to have changes in vision as they age. Dry eye can affect your ability to see clearly; so can "floaters" in the eye. Then if you add other conditions of the eyes, such as cataracts, glaucoma, or macular degeneration, these diseases can cause significant impairment when driving.

A driver can have emotional changes as they age. Sometimes people become more emotional when they drive- becoming more nervous, irritable, or even angry when driving. These emotions can lead to incidents of road rage. Road rage can occur at any time and may reflect important other issues in a person's life, but it may also increase with aging. As one ages they experience diminished cognitive abilities; slower processing skills of the brain, slower reaction time, and slower multi-tasking ability. One can experience impaired short-term memory or even reduced attention span. Have you ever driven somewhere, and arrived at your destination, only to realize that you have no idea how you got there? You got lost in your thoughts and you were not paying attention to your driving to the degree that you should have.

It is common for people to have medical conditions as they age, which can impact driving. And it is important to be aware of medications that may affect driving. It is recommended that you talk to your pharmacist about each new prescription, to determine if it might affect your driving. And that talk should include over the counter medications- these also can impair driving skills.

Financial difficulties may make driving too challenging. It is expensive to purchase a vehicle, maintain the vehicle, purchase insurance and gas. And when a driver has less income, the driver may not be able to afford the privilege of driving. When a driver has a pattern of close calls, the individual may become concerned enough to stop driving on their own, or family/friends may express concern about the individual driving.

Sometimes a driver will lose confidence in their ability to drive. Particularly when you live in a very congested area, it can be challenging to drive. Here in Southern California, there is ongoing construction, heavy commuting times in the morning and evening, and many trucks that travel the freeways. All of these situations can become stressful to an older driver, and they may cease or restrict their driving due to the stressful situations they face.

There are situations where friends or family will express concern about an individual's ability to drive, and a person who recognizes their difficulty with driving might realize the dangers of driving and will stop. And sometimes a driver will have revocation of the driver's license and will stop driving. One gentleman was tested who had his driver's license revoked, and had a California ID. When he was tested for driving, he showed his California ID, and was informed that he did not have a valid driver's license. He argued that he had a valid driver's license, which indicates that he had forgotten he had an accident, had his license revoked, and was taken to the DMV to get his California ID.

And despite only having an ID, he was able to go to a dealership and purchase a brand-new sports car.

Aging is the most significant factor to increase the risk of developing dementia, but dementia is not a normal part of aging. Not knowing one has dementia or being in denial about the effects of dementia can lead to the risk of many older licensed drivers to continued driving even though they are not safe to drive. Drivers living with dementia are at an increased risk of causing traffic accidents. According to a study by Friedland and coworkers there is a 37% increase in rate of crashes of older drivers living with Alzheimer's disease compared to older individuals who are not living with dementia. This study included 30 individuals living with dementia, and 20 age-matched individuals in a control group.

To clarify- not all drivers with dementia are unsafe to drive, particularly in early stages of dementia. That is why a driving assessment is so important- the driver living with dementia must be evaluated to determine the current cognitive functional level and assess whether the individual is still safe to drive. If the individual is determined to be safe to drive, there must be an assessment given on a regular basis to determine continued fitness to drive. It is recommended to have an assessment every six months to a year, depending on the physician's current assessment of cognitive impairment. If the driver is determined to be unsafe to drive, then the Occupational Therapist will report the driver to the state Department of Motor Vehicles and request the driver's license to be revoked.

The question is asked frequently if getting a GPS system is a safe option for older adults, or other features in newer model cars. Research says that the older driver who is cognitively intact can probably learn how to use new technologies effectively, but it will take longer for them to learn than a younger adult driver. While these features may work well with older adults who are cognitively intact, it is likely that they will increase the risk of unsafe driving with individuals who are living with dementia. The first thing to consider for these drivers is the lack of experience with technology. If they have limited or no experience with GPS or other new features in a car, they are unlikely to learn how to use this technology, and it will probably increase the risk of causing an accident, rather than preventing one.

Some older adults can adapt, adjust and compensate for the age-related changes they experience, and learn how to stay safe when driving. It is very important for ALL drivers to avoid multi-tasking when driving, but especially important for older drivers. The older brain is not equipped to multi-task but driving requires the ultimate ability to switch attention rapidly. So, for older adults it is very important to get the heater or air conditioner set, seating and mirrors adjusted, all before starting the car and driving. It is even recommended not to play music while driving. And of course, no cell phone conversations or texting while driving. Conversations with passengers can be a dangerous distraction to an older driver, and drivers have been observed refusing to engage in conversation while driving because they do not want the distraction. Some drivers will create more space for reaction time by driving slower and creating larger distance between vehicles, but these drivers must be mindful of not driving significantly under the speed limit.

In California, one can get a ticket for driving significantly under the speed limit as well as over the speed limit. All drivers must anticipate and plan for unexpected occurrences when driving, and this is especially important for the older driver. Older adults will benefit from exercising regularly to maintain strength, flexibility, coordination, and brain health. In some cases, older adults will restrict their driving to within five miles of the home, only drive during the day or only on sunny days, and often will avoid freeways. One must be mindful that most accidents happen within five miles of home, so restricting distance driving will not, in and of itself, make an older driver safe to drive.

Chapter 3

Health Professional and Family's Role

Driving is often viewed as a right by the older adult population, to complete errands, see the doctor, remain connected to family and friends in the community, purchase groceries and medications, and retain their independence. There are parts of the country that do not have adequate alternatives for maintaining these activities if the individual is no longer safe to drive and does not live with at least one person who can drive. This burden of transportation is often forced on the caregiver, either a family member or paid caregiver. When a family member becomes responsible for transportation, it may curtail their ability to work outside the home, sometimes causing the individual to lose their job. Retiring from driving may cause depression in the individual, and possibly to the caregiver.

The physician can play a critical role in helping the patient decide to retire from driving. Persson conducted an interview study of 56 older adults who stopped driving. He found that 27% decided to retire from driving based on the recommendation of the physician. Most of these individuals stated that it was a personal decision based on recommendations from the physician and family, as well as having medical issues of concern. Other studies for individuals living with dementia revealed the same reasons for retiring from driving,

There was a survey in Connecticut where there were 3,450 physicians interviewed, and 77% responded that they had a conversation with older adult patients regarding driving. This survey also indicates that 23% did not have this discussion with patients. Of the physicians surveyed, 74% stated that there should be some type of screening method for older drivers, and only 59% believed it was their responsibility to report a patient deemed to be an unsafe driver. As of this writing there are only six states that require a physician to report an unsafe driver to the Department of Motor Vehicles. Some are specific about the conditions that should be reported, and others provide limited guidance. Twenty-two states provide limited guidance for reporting, but do not require it. In a study by Adler, Rottunda, and Kuskowski (1999), 46% of licensed drivers who had been diagnosed with Alzheimer's type dementia reported that they were hesitant to retire from driving based solely on the physician's advice. Some states provide confidentiality as well as protection from litigation for physicians who do report unsafe drivers.

Unfortunately, drivers living with dementia often stop driving only after a significant crash. Drachman and other researchers stated that renewing a driver's license for an elderly driver should be based on ability to drive safely rather than simply on a medical diagnosis. The Alzheimer's Association stated, "The diagnosis of Alzheimer's disease is not, on its own, a sufficient reason to withdraw driving privileges. The determining factor in withdrawing driving privileges should be an individual's driving ability."

The confusion about when to retire from driving seems to be most relevant for the individual who has mild to moderate dementia. If an individual has a history of accidents or tickets, and difficulty with visual processing skills, executive function/decisions, or judgment, then a behind-the-wheel assessment is recommended. However, the American

Academy of Neurology published guidelines asserting that an individual with mild dementia should not drive. The question is- do we wait until the individual has multiple accidents before requiring a driving assessment, or should we test an individual diagnosed with dementia at the mild stage?

The recommended factors that a physician should consider when referring for a driving assessment or reporting the individual to the Department of Motor Vehicles should be: severity of the dementia, family report, male gender, and performance on testing including visuospatial skills, executive function, and judgment. Physicians can provide this screening during an office visit, and then refer to a Neuropsychologist for neuropsychological testing, and an Occupational Therapist for driving assessment.

But studies reveal that the physician often has difficulty with ensuring compliance that the patient will stop driving once a physician has recommended cessation. Commonly, the individual living with dementia does not recognize that there is a problem with driving skills, and even if they do recognize a problem the individual often dismisses the physician's concerns- whether the person fears the loss of independence or for other reasons. The family members can help by working on taking away the keys, the car, or other methods as listed in this book. The Alzheimer's Disease Association has published these recommendations: (1) acknowledge the loss, (2) arrange for alternate transportation, (3) solicit the support of others (friends, family, insurance agent), (4) make the car less accessible, (5) require the individual to take a driving test, (6) be firm.

Sometimes an escalated effort is required for individuals living with more advanced dementia who are not willing to comply with voluntary cessation of driving. It is also common knowledge that revoking the license does not stop the individual from driving, especially when the individual has a deficit of judgment and insight. In a case we cited earlier, a man totaled his car in an accident he caused, and his license had been revoked. He went to the dealership and bought a sports car, paying cash for the car. And when we asked to see his driver's license, he showed his California ID. He forgot that his license had been revoked and that he went to the DMV to get the new ID. With this degree of memory loss, it would be dangerous for him to drive, among other reasons, because he might not even be able to find his way home.

As a last resort you can take the car keys or take the vehicle away, but you can only take the vehicle if you have legal power of attorney. The problem with taking the keys is that sometimes the individual has another set of keys hidden away, so you must ensure that all the keys are confiscated. We have been told of numerous individuals with dementia who called the police when the family removed the vehicle and the family did not have the proper legal documents in place. The police informed these individuals they would be arrested if they did not return the vehicle. So, for the family, it is important to get the title to the vehicle changed to include another person while the person living with dementia is still lucid enough and willing to do this.

If you do have the legal documents to remove the car, you can try to remove it to a distant site for "repairs". Sometimes a younger family member needs a car, and the car can be gifted to that individual. If you sell the vehicle, you can use the money from the sale to fund transportation for the affected individual. Another warning: if you disable the car you need to write a note, such as "Dear Mr. Mechanic- please do not fix this car. My loved one has dementia and is no longer safe to drive. Please call me at this number: (xxx) xxx-xxxx".

We acknowledge that there is a great deal of complicated information in this chapter, and we did not address the heavy emotional toll that this takes on the family, and sometimes even the medical professionals who are working with the individual and the family. Know that there are resources to assist you with this difficult transition, and recommendations on how to approach the individual for family, friend, and medical professionals. We also want to acknowledge that there may be other medical providers who may be involved in this process, such as physician's assistants, nurses and nurse practitioners, occupational, physical, and speech therapists.

Chapter 4

Not Normal Aging: Its Effects

The senses normally become more impaired as we age but diseases of the eye can occur including cataracts, macular degeneration, glaucoma, and retinopathy. Cataracts cause blurry, distorted vision, and make night driving even more difficult. Macular degeneration does not affect vision in early stage, but if the disease progresses, people experience wavy or blurred vision, and later stage causes loss of central vision. Glaucoma damages the optic nerve, impairing the ability to send information from the eyes to the brain. The individual with glaucoma will begin to lose patches of vision, usually peripheral vision.

The ears have two jobs- maintain balance, and hearing. While impaired balance can cause difficulty walking to and from the car, it can also cause dizziness, lightheadedness, blurred vision, disorientation, or confusion. All those symptoms can impact a person's ability to drive safely. Loss of hearing can greatly impact a driver's ability to respond to emergency situations. I tested a woman who demonstrated low hearing, and she had been diagnosed with middle stage dementia. Just after I instructed the woman to "Make a left turn at the next signal," an ambulance and fire truck with lights on and sirens blaring started to cross the intersection. The driver continued into the left turn lane and attempted to cross the intersection with the green light. The driving instructor had to step on the brake to prevent an accident. The woman expressed great frustration at being stopped, and I had to explain to her that there were emergency vehicles crossing the intersection and she was required to stop. When we were returning to the driver's home, the same two emergency vehicles were going in the opposite direction, once again she attempted to cross the intersection, and the driving instructor again had to intervene. She did not see and process the visual information of the vehicles and did not hear the sirens from either vehicle. Both decreased sensations impacted her ability to drive safely.

In a study of drivers with hearing impairment, these drivers were less likely to successfully maneuver around road hazards, had a significantly impaired performance when distractions were present, and took more time when attempting to complete the course. Having a diagnosis of dementia, in addition to another sensory impairment, will greatly reduce driving safety. Meniere's disease can cause dulled hearing, vertigo (dizziness with a spinning sensation), tinnitus, ear pressure, and can distort loud noises. These attacks can last from 20 minutes to 4 hours, and most people feel very sleepy after the attack. You can imagine how difficult it would be to attempt driving while feeling dizzy, or become distracted by ringing in the ears, or feel pressure in the ears. Adding cognitive impairment to any of those disorders will intensify the impact on driving.

Touch is another sensation that is necessary for driving. Your foot must be placed in the correct position on the gas and brake pedals. You need to know how much pressure to apply to each pedal, have accurate pressure that is needed for braking or accelerating, and be able to move the foot between the two pedals with adequate reaction time. If a driver has peripheral neuropathy in the right foot, for example, driving will be impaired, and California DMV will not allow individuals to drive with this condition. Having foot drop (the inability to lift the front part of the foot) will also impair the ability to drive safely. Foot drop is caused by paralysis or weakness of the muscles that lift the foot and can be caused by nerve injury, compression of a nerve (such as sciatica), brain and spinal cord disorders such as multiple sclerosis, amyotrophic lateral sclerosis, polio, Charcot-Marie-Tooth disease, or stroke.

There is no such thing as true multi-tasking. The brain is simply shifting focus very quickly. This slows down a great deal with aging. Driving requires constant shifting of focus, and with dementia this ability is significantly diminished. Drivers must pay attention to street signs, signal lights, lines painted on the road, and traffic around the car. We must also remember the state's driving laws. We need to understand the dashboard gauges- the speedometer, the gas level, oil pressure, tire pressure, and if you have GPS- how to get to the destination. If one adds any distraction like turning on the AC or the heat, changing radio stations, talking to a passenger, answering the cell phone while driving- all those tasks are very difficult for the brain to manage in addition to driving. Probably the most important distraction to avoid is texting and driving, with talking on a cell phone coming in as a close second for increasing crash rates. The National Safety Council reported there are 1.6 million crashes each year, causing 390,000 injuries, and 9 people are killed daily, due to distracted driving.

However, there is a significant difference in perception of the dangers of texting and driving when millennials (25-34) are compared to boomers (55-65+). For the millennials, 29.8% believe they are capable of multitasking moderately well, and 20.3% believe they can multi-task extremely well. For the boomers, 33.9% believe that they can multitask moderately well, but only 13.8% believe they can multitask extremely well. The aging brain has much more difficulty with shifting attention quickly- using the cell phone in any capacity while driving will significantly raise the risk of an accident for all drivers, but especially affects older drivers.

Add to this one more important point made: many older adults I've tested have cognitive impairment and drive two footed. Most of these drivers step on the gas pedal and the brake at the same time throughout the drive. Since their sensory perception is impaired and they have cognitive impairment, they are not aware that they are doing this. What are the consequences of this? One foot tends to press harder than the other foot, so the driver may unintentionally but drastically speed up or slow down, depending on the pressure of each foot on the respective pedal. This causes increased errors with accelerating and braking.

The aging brain also needs more information and more time to decide what to do in any given situation. The driver with dementia will have significantly more difficulty with problem solving when driving, especially in new or unfamiliar circumstances. Imagine the driver approaching an intersection and the signal lights have changed format. For example, there are new signal lights in California where there is a green arrow, then a flashing yellow arrow. If the driver has never seen this signal light before, they have limited time to figure out what to do. Can I go on the yellow arrow? Do I slow down or stop at the yellow arrow? Are there cars approaching from the opposite direction? Are they going straight, or turning, or stopping? All these questions must be answered quickly. The aging brain with dementia will have greater difficulty deciding what to do and the driver is much more likely to cause an accident with new or complicated signal lights.

Real World Concerns

If you are a family member with a loved one living with dementia, or you or a professional who works with older adults, these are the areas that you can watch and observe for mistakes that might indicate difficulty with driving:

- Confusion with filling out forms
- Not paying bills, or paying the same bill several times
- Confusion with taking medications correctly
- Visual deficits
- Getting lost when on the way to or coming home from a familiar place
- Difficulty balancing the check book
- New medication (prescribed or over the counter) affecting driving

Real World Concerns Cont.

- Compromised physical status- difficulty with walking or getting in and out of the car

- Coordination problems

- Family member or friend's concern after observing difficulty in daily tasks

Chapter 5

Mild Cognitive Impairment

The term Mild Cognitive Impairment or MCI was originally coined by Dr. Barry Reisberg in 1982. Since then MCI has been extensively studied and the diagnostic criteria steadily refined. MCI is a syndrome of cognitive decline greater than expected for an individual's age and education level, but one that does not meet the diagnostic criteria for dementia. The cognitive changes (deficits) in memory, language, visual processing ability, or executive function are severe enough to be noticeable to other people and to show up on tests of cognitive functioning. However, these changes are not severe enough to significantly interfere with the person's everyday social and occupational functioning. This is what distinguishes this cognitive disorder from dementia.

- Dr. Ron Peterson and his colleagues at the Mayo Clinic have developed the core diagnostic criteria for MCI. It is as follows:

1. A memory complaint- preferably corroborated by a family member or caregiver

2. Objective memory impairment for the person's age (ideally confirmed by neuropsychological testing)

3. Normal general cognitive function

4. Ability to perform activities of daily living

5. No dementia

6. May also include irritability, depression, apathy, aggression, and anxiety

These might include any of the following:

- Asking the same questions repeatedly

- Telling the same stories repeatedly

- Forgetting the name of major streets surrounding the home

- Getting lost when attempting to drive to/from familiar places

- Forgetting recent conversations

- Unusual bouts of anger or road rage while driving

- Frequently misplacing belongings

- Refusing to drive with others in the car

- Not remembering names of familiar people

- Not getting services needed for the car

- Forgetting that something is cooking on the stove

- Forgetting to pay bills or paying bills more than once

- Forgetting appointments or forgetting to take medications

- No longer doing things like reading novels or playing Bridge, because memory is impaired

- Difficulty learning a new device (cell phone, TV remote, computer)

Vascular Cognitive Impairment

- Mild cognitive deficits-result of stroke or vascular disease
- Deficit or deficits not severe enough to significantly impact everyday social and occupational functioning

- Do not meet the full diagnostic criteria for Vascular Dementia

Clinical Vignette: Mrs. Johnson was a 67-year-old retired woman with a one-year history of memory problems. She reported that her memory was worse than a few years prior and the symptoms were accelerating. She said she had to write everything down on Post-It Notes and put them all over her house. She also complained of some word-finding difficulty, which she said was a new development. Her husband reported that, indeed, there has been a definite and persistent change in her memory and language abilities compared to her previous level of cognitive functioning five years earlier. However, Mrs. Johnson denied that the problems significantly interfered with her everyday social and occupational functioning. She said she could still drive but has been getting confused and even lost in familiar areas. She could still pay their bills, manage their finances, cook all the meals, go shopping alone and even travel alone across country by plane to visit their daughter

Chapter 6

Dementia

What is dementia? The word *dementia* means literally from Latin "to lose one's mind." Dementia is a general term for a group of brain disorders. In medical terms it is a syndrome meaning a collection of signs and symptoms that tend to occur together. It is an umbrella term used to describe any significant and persistent decline in cognitive function.

In 1900 there were fewer than three million people over the age of 65 in the United States. At the time of this writing there are about 40 million, and this number is expected to double by the year 2050. Age is the number one risk factor for dementia and Mild Cognitive Impairment with 95% of all cases of Alzheimer's dementia occurring over the age of 65.

Dementia is a neurological disorder characterized by the loss of cognitive abilities including memory, language skills, reasoning ability, abstract thinking, spatial ability and orientation along with personality and behavioral changes. It is caused by brain damage resulting from an event such as a traumatic brain injury or a stroke, or from a progressive disease such as Alzheimer's disease. The parts of the brain that are most affected are the association areas of the brain, which integrate sensory information, thought, memory, and purposeful behavior. When extensive damage to these areas occurs, the affected person will begin showing cognitive deficits, mild at first and gradually becoming more severe.

There are over 70 different causes for dementia- some are reversible but most are irreversible. Most dementias begin gradually (months to years) as with Alzheimer's disease or vascular dementia. It may also begin suddenly as after a major stroke or traumatic brain injury. The symptoms of dementia may be reversible as when the cause is a medication side effect or a correctible medical condition such as a thyroid disorder. Other potentially reversible causes include infections, toxins, nutritional deficiencies, metabolic disturbances, and even psychiatric conditions such as major depression. However, most types of dementia are non-reversible and progressive such as with Alzheimer's disease. It is worth noting that Alzheimer's disease is only one- although the most common- type of dementia. In other words, a person with dementia may or may not have Alzheimer's disease, but a person with Alzheimer's disease always has dementia.

Types of Dementia:

- Dementia of the Alzheimer's type (60 to 75%)

- Dementia due to Creutzfeldt-Jacob disease

- Frontotemporal Dementia (Pick's Disease) (5-8%)

- Vascular Dementia (5 to 10%)

- Dementia due to Head Trauma

- Dementia due to Huntington's disease

- Dementia with Lewy Bodies (10 to 20%)

- Dementia due to HIV disease

- Dementia due to Parkinson's disease

- Alcohol-Induced Persisting Dementia

While there are many causes for the symptoms of dementia, Alzheimer's disease, Lewy Body disease, frontotemporal lobar degeneration, and vascular disease account for over 95% of all dementias. Recent studies are showing that many, if not most, people with dementia have more than one cause for the dementia. An example is a combination of Alzheimer's disease and Vascular disease.

Potentially Reversible Causes of Dementia

- Emotional distress or depression

- Nutritional deficiencies

- Metabolic disturbances

- Infections (encephalitis, meningitis, etc.)

- Reactions to medications

- Normal pressure hydrocephalus (partially reversible)

- Endocrine abnormalities (e.g. thyroid dysfunction)

- Brain tumor

Hearing impairment can be mistaken for memory loss. Evaluating a person's hearing can be a necessary step in testing them.

Chapter 7

Alzheimer's Disease (AD)

- Discovered in 1906 by a German psychiatrist/ neuropathologist Dr. Alois Alzheimer (1864-1915)

- Auguste Deter, 51-year-old

- Symptoms: depression, paranoia, delusions, and dementia

- She died in 1906 at age 55

- Dr. Alzheimer recognized signs and symptoms from a new disease process that had not been previously described in the literature

- Used recently developed staining techniques to examine brain tissue under a microscope

- Identified amyloid plaque and neurofibrillary tangles

- Now most cases of Alzheimer's dementia (95%) occur over the age of 65

Alzheimer's Disease Symptoms

- Multiple cognitive deficits

-Affects both memory and cognition

1. Memory impairment- difficulty with learning new information or ability to recall previously learned information

2. One or more of these:

   - Aphasia (The loss of ability to understand or express speech)

   - Apraxia (The inability to perform learned – or familiar – movements on command)

   - Agnosia (The incapacity to interpret sensations and hence to recognize things)

   - Impairment in executive functioning (The struggle with multitasking, working memory, self-control, problem-solving, and planning)

These deficits can cause significant impairment in social or occupational   functioning and will certainly have a negative impact on driving.

   - Gradual onset

   - Continuing cognitive decline

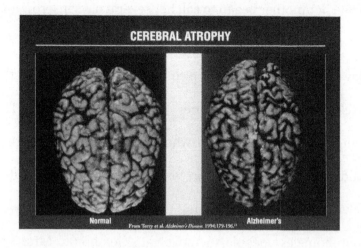

This photo is an example of the significant loss of brain volume and function when affected by Alzheimer's. Neurons become injured and die, the connections between the neurons are broken down. Many regions of the brain begin to shrink.

Clinical Vignette: Mrs. Lee, a 68-year-old woman, had been living alone in her home in Laguna Beach, California, for the past 10 years since her husband died. She had been a very successful businesswoman who always showed good judgment in everything she did. She had one daughter who lived and worked in San Francisco. They saw each other two to three times a year but spoke on the phone several times a week. Mrs. Lee always said that everything was fine, and she was having no problems. The daughter became concerned when her mother began to call her several days in a row and ask the same question or tell the same story she had told the day before. The daughter also began to hear voices in the background every time they spoke on the phone. The daughter asked her mother who was there, and her mother said they were just neighbors visiting. The daughter decided to visit her mother. She found that her mother had allowed four homeless people to move into her home. Mrs. Lee explained that in return for living in her home they would help with the cleaning, cooking, shopping, and paying her bills. Mrs. Lee felt this was all quite reasonable. The daughter was understandably shocked and brought her mother to see her primary care physician who diagnosed Mrs. Lee with early Alzheimer's disease.

Chapter 8

Lewy Body Dementia (LBD)

- Dr. Frederick Lewy discovered the abnormal microscopic deposits- referred to as Lewy bodies

- Dr. Lewy worked at the Neuropsychiatric Laboratory in Berlin, Germany

- He emigrated to the U.S. in 1934, and changed his name to Frederic Henry Lewey

- Lewy Body Dementia produces cognitive decline

- Patients fluctuate in terms of attention, alertness, and ability to speak coherently

- Also called Dementia with Lewy Bodies

- Progressive dementia characterized by:

  - Features of Alzheimer's disease (impaired short-term memory)

  - Features of Parkinson's disease: tendency to fall, bradykinesia (slowed movement), rigidity, postural instability, shuffling gait, akinesia (loss of ability to move arms/legs voluntarily)

- Fluctuating levels of alertness
- Intermittent delirium (reduced awareness of surroundings, confused thinking, emotional disruptions)
- Delusions- disconnection with reality, fixed belief that is not true (e.g. belief that one is being watched through the TV)
- <u>Detailed</u> visual hallucinations early stage of the disease- seeing something that isn't there (e.g. aliens landed a spacecraft in the front yard)
- Adverse reaction to antipsychotic medications (Risperidone, Olanzapine, Seroquel)
- Sleep disturbance may be present (may physically act out dreams, may kick or hit spouse)
- Course is more rapid than with AD
- Progressive cognitive decline
- Slowed movements
- Significant decline in social or occupational functioning; memory loss may occur later

Example of driving impairment: One 66 year-old-woman with this diagnosis stated that she was forced to stop driving by her family because she was hallucinating cars and trucks driving through the windshield toward her head. She started causing accidents in her panic to avoid these hallucinations. She further stated that her husband did not like to drive with her in the car, because she continued to have these same hallucinations, and every time she "saw" a vehicle driving through the windshield, she would scream and grab her husband's arm.

Chapter 9

Frontotemporal Dementia (FTD)/Pick's Disease

- Dr. Arnold Pick (1581-1924)

  - A neurologist from the Czech Republic- the first to describe a patient with FTD

- Unknown cause, slow progression

- Produces atrophy primarily of the frontal lobes of the brain

- Insidious, with prominent changes in personality- increased apathy and loss of empathy

- Memory loss and difficulty with language

- Memory, figure-copying, and calculations are largely spared until middle stages of the disease

- Early signs of disinhibition

- Initially don't show memory impairment

- Usually will perform normally on all commonly used dementia screening instruments (e.g. MMSE, MMSE-2, MoCA)

- Depression, anxiety

- Often misdiagnosed for months or years before a correct diagnosis is made

There are three subtypes of FTD:

1. **Behavioral variant FTD (bvFTD)**

   - Can occur in people in 50s or 60s
   - Personality and behavioral changes - disinhibition, impulsiveness, tactlessness, and impaired social judgment (in some cases extreme apathy)
   - Pick's disease is the most common type.

2. **Primary Progressive Aphasia (PPA)**

   Changes in:

   - Language skills
   - Writing and speaking
   - Comprehension
   - Semantic- lose ability to understand or formulate words

- Non-fluent: speech is hesitant, ungrammatical, or labored

Clinical Vignette: The following actual case was taken from a 2008 newspaper article written by the man's wife. Mr. Kalmash, was a 60 year old man, who began showing symptoms ten years earlier. There were very noticeable changes over time. His wife said that her husband began showing significant personality changes. He had become selfish and self-centered. He lacked emotion and empathy. He began displaying compulsive behaviors and quirky habits, all of which were new. His judgment was poor, and he was showing poor impulse control. He had had a lucrative job as a sales and marketing director for over 16 years until he came home one day in 2006 with a six-page letter explaining why he was being fired. The letter described all the things he had not been doing on his job. The wife reported that after consulting with sixteen physicians, four of whom were neurologists, they still did not have a correct diagnosis. It is noteworthy that Mr. Kalmash had no memory or language problems at that time. It was only after being evaluated by specialists at The Brain and Aging Institute at UC Irvine that a correct diagnosis was obtained. Mr. Kalmash was diagnosed with Frontotemporal

Dementia. Following this his condition continued to deteriorate until he was forced to go into a board and care facility where he received 24-hour assistance. He later developed difficulty walking and aphasia, but as far as his wife and doctors could tell Mr. Kalmash had no significant memory impairment. The fact that he had no memory impairment early on, and yet his condition further deteriorated, made it difficult for the earlier evaluators to recognize this as a progressive dementing disorder.

Chapter 10

Vascular Dementia (VaD)

- Caused by vascular disease
- Chronic low blood flow to the brain (vascular insufficiency) due to blocked arteries or stenosis, cerebral hemorrhage, thrombosis, or embolism
- Brain cell loss- also called a cerebrovascular accident (CVA)
- 25% of major strokes produce some degree of dementia
- Multiple small strokes can also produce cognitive deficits, MCI and dementia
- Presence of a dementia syndrome
- Symptoms not occurring exclusively during the course of delirium

Case Vignette: Mrs. Lawson, a 67-year-old woman, was admitted to a rehabilitation unit following seven days on the medical floor for treatment of a major stroke. The stroke involved her left hemisphere and subsequently resulted in mild to moderate speech impairment along with moderate memory impairment. Once it was clear that the initial delirium had resolved, she underwent a thorough neuropsychological evaluation. Test results were consistent with a diagnosis of dementia. The family was interviewed to obtain relevant history about her premorbid cognitive functioning. They reported that Mrs. Lawson had no cognitive deficits at all prior to the stroke. She was able to drive, pay bills, manage the family finances, manage her medications, and go shopping on her own without difficulty. She had even traveled alone across the country to attend her college reunion a few weeks before the stroke. Prior to the stroke she played Bridge every week and was attending college classes to learn Spanish. Based upon the chronology of the stroke and the onset of the patient's significant cognitive deficits, the etiology of her dementia was determined to be the stroke. Her diagnosis was Vascular Dementia.

Chapter 11

How Cognitive Abilities are Assessed

It is important for a person to have a thorough assessment if there is a question about cognitive abilities such as memory or decision making skills, ability to perform self-care tasks, or ability to perform normal day-today activities such as paying bills and managing finances. In two studies, one by SE Lesikar and associates, the other by GK Fox and associates, the conclusion was the Mini-Mental State Examination (MMSE) was not accurate in predicting future crashes or traffic violations among older adults. The MMSE is a brief cognitive measure focusing on memory, language, and orientation, and was not created to assess driving ability. The Neuropsychological Assessment Battery was created as a tool for evaluating visual processing skills related to driving in individuals living with dementia. The results of this test correlated with behind-the-wheel performance in individuals who were deemed healthy and for those with mild dementia. A meta-analysis of literature involving neuropsychological testing compared to safe driving abilities supported the need for testing visual processing skills to predict the individual's ability to drive safely. This was compared to testing results of other cognitive functions, including language, memory, and attention. The section of testing that was most relevant to driving abilities were the visual processing skills- what the driver can see, process, and then respond appropriately. It is interesting that memory tests did not directly correlate to driving abilities in a person living with dementia, according to the studies.

Clinical Vignette

During the process of a driving assessment of an 85-year-old female, who was a retired Vice President of a real estate company, she scored 23/30 on the SLUMS (St. Louis University Mental Status Exam). Her memory was fair- she scored 70% on one of the memory subtests, 75% on another subtest, 100% on the last subtest. During the driving portion of the test, she mixed up the gas and brake pedals, slowed down at a green light, had difficulty keeping the car in the correct lane position, switched lanes without looking to determine if it was safe to change lanes, drove through a red light, did not stop for a pedestrian crossing in front of the car- she kept driving toward the pedestrian while he walked across the street, and started to enter a lane that was occupied by another car because she wanted the driver to get out of her way. All of these mistakes required intervention of the driving instructor.

Driving Simulator Testing

There is a trend now to provide driving assessments with a driving simulator, and not a behind-the-wheel test. In a study by Cox and colleagues, an interactive driving simulator was used to evaluate an individual's driving performance. They compared drivers living with dementia to a similarly aged control group with the use of a driving simulator and found that the individuals with a dementia diagnosis more often drove under the speed limit, drove off the road, had more difficulty with left hand turns, and had difficulty with applying the correct brake pressure when stopping. In another study utilizing a simulator, researchers conducting a study using the Iowa Driving Simulator hypothesized that drivers with dementia had poor visual attention which caused increased crashes. The researchers created potential crash scenarios where opposing traffic would make an illegal maneuver at an intersection. The individuals who "crashed" proved that they lacked adequate attention or demonstrated slow or inappropriate responses to the scenarios. It may be important, according to neuropsychological research, that the most important tests related to ability to drive safely are executive function and visuospatial ability. Executive function requires the ability to manage complex tasks while driving, ability to pay attention to the road and possible hazards, surrounding traffic, appropriate driving skills for the circumstances, and filter relevant and irrelevant information while driving.

Mild Cognitive Impairment (MCI)

Individuals diagnosed with MCI may demonstrate potentially dangerous changes in their ability to drive safely, even though MCI is not a diagnosis of dementia, because driving requires highly complex skills that require the ability to integrate cognition, visuospatial, and motor function abilities. If a driver has a diagnosis of multidomain MCI they are more likely to demonstrate difficulty with adequate memory, executive function, and visuospatial skills well before they demonstrate difficulty with self-care tasks such as bathing, dressing, or toileting. If they have difficulty in these areas, they are likely to have difficulty remembering the meaning of signal lights and traffic signs, increased difficulty with being able to find their way to familiar places, difficulty making a quick decision when faced with an emergency situation, or seeing and processing what they need to do while driving. It is also likely that they will have a compromised response to any changes in their usual area of driving such as construction or repaving projects. Likewise, they are apt to have more difficulty responding appropriately if another driver makes an erratic, unexpected move.

A driver with MCI may also process incoming information more slowly, which leads to slower reaction time. It will be difficult for the individual to make quick decisions when driving due to weak or impaired judgment. However, the family or doctor may not see any problems in their judgment when performing daily tasks at home or during a routine medical exam.

Short-term memory is usually impaired with MCI, so the driver may forget the destination they selected prior to leaving home or forget why they wanted to go to the grocery store. In testing a driver with short term memory impairment, the driver will attempt to remember the destination they were asked to reach and will try to cover up the mistake. They either continue to drive to a random destination because they forgot the destination, or sometimes will admit they made a mistake and ask for help to remember the destination. This is different than a response from a driver who has been diagnosed with dementia. Their response, instead, is to randomly drive around and point out landmarks they are familiar with or begin to drive home because of they can't remember the chosen destinations. They typically make more driving errors at this point because of the increased anxiety of forgetting the destination they created.

Attention span with MCI will become weak or impaired, which can lead to more mistakes as drivers try to cope with normal challenges in addition to attempting to multi-task. These becomes a monumental challenge for a driver with dementia. Executive functions will be impaired, which leads to difficulties making quick decisions, planning the route, or finding a new address. We have seen people who would drive to a new doctor's office the day before their appointment, just so they would know how to get there and not get lost and miss the appointment. Multi-tasking skills are essential for safe driving, but are abnormally impaired with MCI, and are severely impaired when diagnosed with dementia. The driver with MCI will also have difficulty switching their focus from one type of stimuli to another. They may get distracted by something other than the road and stop focusing on the traffic ahead or the approach to a signal light. This distraction increases dramatically with a diagnosis of dementia.

Dementia

Dementia will have a more significant impact on driving. The driver living with dementia will have a dramatically slower speed of information processing. Reaction time is greatly decreased because the brain influenced by dementia cannot take in all the data the eyes can see, process that information, and then respond with the corrective action. An individual living with dementia has decreased judgment, which can lead to such mistakes as attempting a left-hand turn with oncoming traffic, running through a red light or stop sign, or stopping at a green light. Short term memory is impaired, so the driver can forget where they were headed, or get distracted by conversation in the car and not pay attention to driving.

The individual's executive function will be impaired, which can cause difficulty with making good decisions when driving or planning how to accomplish all the tasks needed to be completed for the day. We talked to a paramedic who was at the scene of an accident and the older female driver told him that she did what she "always", when changing lanes, she would turn on her signal light, count to 10, then switch lanes. She just assumed that all drivers around her would comply with her signal.

When multitasking is impaired the driver will have difficulty paying attention to the gauges in the car and anticipating what to do at intersections. They will have reduced awareness of surrounding traffic, and have difficulty understanding what to do at intersections with multiple lights. They will have difficulty shifting focus quickly, particularly when something unexpected happens. This would include such actions as a driver in front of them braking suddenly, when attempting to back out of a parking space with an oncoming car, or a pedestrian walking across the street who they initially did not see. There is so much that we must pay attention to when we drive. For the brain significantly impaired by dementia, it becomes impossible to manage all this information.

It is important for family members and members of the medical community to be aware of the dangers of an individual driving with dementia. The individual living with dementia is usually not aware that their driving is significantly impaired, and they do not typically stop driving without intervention from family or the medical community.

Chapter 12

Driving is a privilege, not a right

As an Occupational Therapist, I was trained to evaluate an individual's ADLs (Activities of Daily Living), and IADLs (Instrumental Activities of Daily Living). Driving is considered an IADL, and this task will be impaired as a result of living with a diagnosis of dementia. And it is probably the most dangerous impairment because it can impact so many people- not just the driver living with dementia.

One of the issues that needs attention is the individual's belief system regarding driving. Drivers often say, "I've been driving since I was 10 years old, living on the farm, and driving a tractor." Or, "I've been driving more than 70 years. Why do I have to stop driving now?" What these individuals don't understand is that driving is a privilege- not a right. The age of the driver is not the most important criteria for driving-- we must demonstrate the ability to drive safely and to follow state driving laws. We are not entitled to drive- we must demonstrate safe driving or retire from driving.

The deadliest incident that I know of happened when 86-year-old George Weller, who had been diagnosed with a cardiac condition and probably had dementia, in 2003 drove his car through the farmer's market in Santa Monica, California. He killed 10 people and injured 70 pedestrians. Witnesses reported they did not see brake lights on his car throughout his drive through the market. Prior to this incident, he had at least one minor crash and multiple incidents of denting neighbors' garage doors and cars, but had never been reported to the DMV for his impaired driving habits or medical condition. The cause of this accident was probably confusion with mixing up the gas and brake pedals, which is a common mistake for an individual living with dementia.

There are alternative transportation options in some communities, and certainly in larger cities, but not nearly what we need. Many seniors want to continue their lifestyle as they age- their ability to continue participating in activities they enjoy in the community. When one retires, most people want to stay connected to friends and family, most want to carry on meaningful activities such as shopping for groceries and other essentials, visit a senior center, attend church or synagogue, participate in community events. Although community mobility includes various methods of transportation such as buses, taxis, subway (in some areas), Uber and Lyft, driving is still a preferred method of mobility for most licensed adults (Dickerson, Brown Meuel, Ridenour, & Cooper, 2014). Many view community mobility as "a basic human need, and necessary for health, well-being, and quality of life" (Dickerson et al., 2007, p. 578).

Driver's license laws initially required a driver to be a minimum of 18 years, but with the laws that were passed by the 1940s most states required a driver to be a minimum of age 16 to get a driver's license. Most older adults have more experience than other drivers, and they feel they are entitled to drive because of their years of experience. So, if a driver is 86 and has been driving for 70 years, their reasoning is typically, no need to take the driver's license away because of the years of experience with driving. That reasoning does not account for acquired medical conditions or injuries that impair the ability to drive safely. It is rare for an individual living with dementia to give up driving. So the burden then falls on family members, friends, or healthcare professionals to monitor these drivers.

Physicians are mandated reporters in California, and part of their legal duties is to report to the California Department of Public Health when they have diagnosed a patient with dementia. In a study on whether physicians report patients with cognitive impairment to the DPH, most of the physicians interviewed stated that they were aware of the California law, but most stated that they do not report. Physicians have also stated that they do not feel confident in testing a patient in the office for driving safety. They generally have limited time with each patient and do not know what tests to use for screening their patients for impaired driving. The American Medical Association published a guideline for physicians to use for an in-office assessment, but then removed the guideline from the web site due to protests from physicians. The physicians complained because of their need to address medical issues with patients they lacked the time to adequately address driving issues.

This is one of the areas where the role of an Occupational Therapist becomes particularly important, because individuals with cognitive impairment need to be tested behind-the-wheel for driving safety, and occupational therapists can get special training to become qualified to make a determination whether the individual is safe to drive, needs additional driving lessons, or needs to retire from driving. When the physician refers the patient to an occupational therapy driving assessment program, the physician can maintain their relationship with the patient and will not have to report the patient to the Department of Motor Vehicles, since the occupational therapist will submit the driving assessment results to the DMV. The occupational therapist then becomes the "bad guy" in giving the patient the news that they are no longer safe to drive, and the physician is off the hook.

One of the issues that needs attention is the individual's belief system regarding driving. We have often heard, "I've been driving since I was 10 years old, living on the farm, and driving a tractor." Or, "I've been driving more than 60 years. Why do I have to stop driving now?" It is difficult to reason with a person who has dementia, so giving them reasons to stop driving does not typically work. That is why providing a driving assessment is so important. The testing provides an unbiased view of the driving, with concrete reasons to stop driving if that is the case.

All states accept reports of unsafe drivers from physicians, but not all states require physicians to report drivers who have medical conditions or functional impairments that may affect safe driving ability to the state motor vehicle agency. In states without mandatory physician reporting, it is the responsibility of the patient to inform the licensing agency. Do you think that a person living with dementia would voluntarily report themselves? Probably not.

Two of the important issues here, then, are to recognize what skills are necessary for a driver to have in order to drive safely, and how dementia affects these skills/abilities. The California DMV has recently created additional guidelines for dementia and driving. "Dementia is an organic brain disorder characterized by impaired cognition involving memory and judgment. Paranoia and disturbances of higher cortical function are common. Changes in personality and behavior frequently occur."

"Dementia is generally a progressive disorder which passes through stages of mild to moderate to severe. Only drivers with dementia in the mild stage may still have preserved cognitive functions necessary to safely operate a motor vehicle. The department may receive a report of dementia from a variety of sources, including physicians, law enforcement agencies, and relatives of the driver. Regardless of the source of the information (form or letter), the department must follow up by sending the reported driver a Driver Medical Evaluation, except in situations where an immediate action is taken. An action will not be taken by the department against the driving privilege without receiving information from a physician. If the driver fails to submit the required medical information, the driving privilege will be suspended pursuant to Vehicle Code Section 13801."

"Reexamination is only appropriate for drivers whose dementia is still diagnosed as mild. Drivers with a medical diagnosis of moderate to severe dementia need no further testing because progression of the disease beyond the mild stage of dementia renders the person unsafe to drive."

According to the California DMV:

"**Mild Dementia**: The capacity for independent living, including adequate personal hygiene and judgment, remains relatively intact. Work or social activities are, however, significantly impaired. Cognitive skills necessary for safe driving, including attention, [speed of information processing], judgment, and memory, may be significantly impaired. All drivers who have been referred to the department or diagnosed with mild dementia are scheduled for a driver safety reexamination interview. If the driving test was satisfactory, a reexamination is scheduled requiring the driver to return to the department within 6 to 12 months so that the dementia can be reassessed, since a mild stage of dementia can rapidly progress to moderate of severe.

Moderate: Independent living is hazardous, and some degree of supervision is necessary. The individual is unable to adequately cope with the environment. Appropriate interpretation of what is seen may be significantly impaired, causing poor or delayed judgment and reaction. Driving would be dangerous.

Severe: Activities of daily living are so impaired that continual supervision is required, e.g., unable to maintain minimal personal hygiene; largely incoherent or mute. The individual is mentally and physically incapacitated." [These drivers have been somewhat incapacitated since the first stage of dementia]

Important Points to Consider:

The procedure for evaluating the person's fitness for driving safely is straightforward. The problems are the person's willingness to be evaluated and the cost of the evaluation.

Not surprisingly most individuals living with dementia do not want their driving to be tested for safety; they are generally adamant that they are still safe to drive. Once reported to the DMV, however, they do not have a choice. Another barrier to providing testing to these individuals is the expense of the private assessment, not by the DMV, which is typically paid by the individual and not covered by medical or auto insurance. And if the individual does not recognize their impaired driving, why should they spend the money for a driving assessment? It is my opinion that it would be cost effective for insurance companies, both health and car insurance, to cover the cost of the driving assessment. It would be less expensive for these companies to pay for the test and prevent accidents than to pay for the cost of repairing cars or restoring the individual's health after the fact.

Doctors are mandated reporters in some states but commonly prefer not to report patients to the Department of Motor Vehicles to maintain a relationship with the patient.

It is possible to lose the right to drive more abruptly. Sometimes a police officer will conduct a traffic stop, and during the stop will impound the car and take the driver's license as well. If the driver feels this was unjustified, it is important to evaluate the incident- for both the police officer's and the driver's decisions. As in the story told earlier of the man who accused the police officer of ageism. He made an illegal left turn but was completely unaware that it was an illegal turn. He stated that he was humiliated by the officer taking his license and impounding his car. What a sad and traumatic ending to his driving, because he did not stop driving until he was forced to stop by a police officer.

If my loved one is diagnosed with dementia, do they have to stop driving immediately? The simple answer is that the driver must have the skills and ability to drive safely, and if they do not have the capability to drive safely, they need to stop driving. But getting them to stop driving can be difficult and complex. Does the individual have other diseases or medical conditions that may impair their ability to drive safely? Does the individual know they are making driving mistakes? Are they able to correct the mistakes when confronted? Making alternate arrangements for them to continue the same activities such as shopping, getting to doctors' appointments, etc. need to be in place to help them give up driving. It is frequently an arduous ordeal. Driving cessation is a very delicate subject and it does not help to be forceful or condescending to your loved one. If you are concerned about the driving skills, call your loved one's doctor and express concern. If you don't have legal rights to talk with the doctor, you can still give the doctor information about your loved one's driving. Realize, however, that the doctor will not be able to give you feedback on your report. Doctors cannot violate HIPAA laws, but they can listen to information you share regarding your loved one's driving.

Chapter 13

How Dementia
Affects Driving and Reasoning

If the driver takes any medications, the family should check with the pharmacist for possible side effects that may impact driving. Many people who are taking strong pain medications state that these medications do not impair their ability to drive safely. Dementia impacts decision making and self-awareness, and some medications can intensify the symptoms of dementia. It is important to watch the individual as they walk, stand up, sit down, get in and out of a car, and observe if they are having difficulty with these movements. If a person has difficulty with walking and shuffles their feet, for example, or cannot lift their right foot to step up on a curb, that person is likely going to have difficulty with picking up the right foot and moving quickly and accurately between the gas pedal and the brake.

I tested one gentleman who was referred because of family members' concerns. During the assessment, he stated that he enjoyed driving to Laughlin frequently because he liked to gamble. I asked how he reached the casino, which was several hours' drive away, given that he made many mistakes on the driving assessment. He stated, "I always put the cruise control at 80 mph, get in the fast lane, and it's a straight shot to Laughlin". Another aspect of the impact of dementia on this driver is that he "loaned" thousands of dollars to his much younger girlfriend when they were gambling. She asked him for a loan on every trip, but never repaid the money.

While sometimes the individual will express concern about their driving, it is more common for the family to initially be concerned when cognitive impairment is involved. Individuals with cognitive impairment lose their ability to self-regulate with driving, and many times, also their awareness that they have impaired decision-making skills in general. For example, one 83 year-old-woman kept scraping her car on the posts of the carport every time she entered and exited. Her solution was to move the posts out three feet. I suspected that she had cognitive impairment because her solution was to move the carport posts, rather than stop driving. She was a very short person and mentioned in the interview that she has a very high bed, and reported she had difficulty getting into bed. When I asked how she was able to get in and out of her bed, she stated that she would take a running start from the hallway and jump onto her bed. These two situations demonstrate that she had impaired reasoning. Instead of not driving anymore, she moved the carport posts. (I insisted that she make the bed transfers safe by having a handyman cut off the bottom of the posts, so the bed would be the right height for her.) After providing the driving assessment, I had to advise her to stop driving, confirming my initial suspicion that she was no longer safe to drive.

It is important to understand that dementia can impair a driver's decision-making skills in other aspects of their lives, which can impact more than their driving skills. I tested a gentleman who lived in a large retirement community. He made many mistakes- more than any driver I have tested. When we returned to his home, his adult son and daughter were waiting for us. They asked for a report, so I began to read the list of mistakes he made during the driving portion of the assessment. He became increasingly angry at me and started to shout and curse at me. I stopped reading the list, but his son insisted that I finish the list. The gentleman stopped me once again and said there was a woman in the neighborhood that he wanted to date, that he would not take her out in a taxi, and therefore he needed to drive. We had a brief discussion about options, but he disagreed with all options, so I returned to reading my list. The gentleman became even more angry and eventually launched into a cursing tirade at me. His son told me that I did not have to listen to the tirade and requested that I leave.

Two weeks later the daughter called me and stated that I saved her family's life. I asked how I did that, and she explained. She said that his father's car had a recall, but the car was never repaired due to her father having dementia and he did not take it to the dealership to be fixed. When the son was leaving his father's home with his car, the car caught on fire. He jumped out of the car, burning his hands in the process. She stated that members of her family had been driving and riding in that car during visits to her father. She said that if the car had caught on fire when her father or the family members were in the car, they never would have gotten out in time.

I urge family members to report concerns to the physician. It is helpful to medical professionals when a family member speaks up and expresses their concern about the person's driving ability, because it is easier to broach the subject with the individual when the physician has specific information about the person's driving habits.

But it is a problem when the family member protests their loved one being asked to stop driving, because they don't want to be burdened with the responsibility of taking Mom or Dad to the grocery store, the doctor's office, the pharmacy, the hairdresser, and all the other errands that are part of everyday living. When the family is hesitant or resistant to taking on the associated responsibilities, it is much harder to convince the individual that they need to stop driving.

Chapter 14

Research on Driving and Dementia

According to a study published in 2000 by David B. Carr, MD and Brian R. Ott, MD, about 4% of drivers over the age of 75 years have a dementia diagnosis. There are over 5.8 million Americans living with dementia and it is estimated now that 30-40% still drive. Just let that sink in. We understand that older adults want to drive- they like the independence to go where they want to go, when they want to go. After all, we are the nation that guarantees freedom and independence, right? They may need the independence or believe that they do. The problem is that people who are driving with dementia often have no clue that they are unsafe to drive, and do not typically retire from driving without intervention from family or medical professionals. The other major problem that we face is that an individual with cognitive impairment, whether MCI (Mild Cognitive Impairment) or dementia, can have impaired driving, even in early stages, and will be guaranteed to have impaired driving by moderate stage dementia. But it is not common knowledge to doctors and other medical professionals, or to the public, that allowing a person with cognitive impairment to drive may be a risk for not only the driver, but all pedestrians and other drivers near the impaired driver. We do know that all drivers with dementia will become too impaired to drive, but it is possible for some people with early stage cognitive impairment to continue driving and may never get to the stage of not being safe to drive. It is impossible to predict if or when the person with simple cognitive impairment will become so impaired that they are no longer safe to drive. So how do we make that determination?

According to SeniorDriving.AAA.com, drivers over the age of 75 have the highest collision rates per distance driven, even if the individual has restricted their own driving. If you add cognitive impairment or a type of dementia such as Alzheimer's disease, the risk of collision is 2.5 to 4.7 greater when compared to healthy, age-matched individuals, according to American Automobile Association. Even drivers with mild dementia have increased risk of diminished safety awareness during an on-road driving assessment. Among other problems, a common mistake I've seen on the driving portion of the test is that drivers with dementia often fail to demonstrate an appropriate response to hazards on the road, increasing risk of causing an accident.

There has been an ongoing debate among medical professionals as to how the driving performance should be evaluated. What is the most accurate way to assess whether a driver with cognitive impairment is safe or unsafe to drive? Each state has a motor vehicle department that uses a number system to determine if unsafe driving behaviors are present. A study by Rachel W Jones Ross, MSc, Charles Scialfa PhD, and Sheila T.D. Cordazzo, PhD asserted that this approach does not delineate the difference between common driving errors and more hazardous errors that might indicate a significant decline in driving safety, so they created an on-road performance assessment of healthy older adults, focusing on these three areas: hazardous infractions, total points accumulated, and comprehensive pass-fail assessments.

They used the Roadwise Review from AAA and the hazard perception test, along with other tests to determine which combination of tests had the most predictive validity. During the first of two sessions they tested participants for contrast sensitivity, visual acuity, and color vision. In the second session they used the MMSE (Mini Mental Status Exam) and the Roadwise Review. The Roadwise Review has eight subtests that appear in this order: leg strength and general mobility, head and neck flexibility, high-contrast visual acuity, low-contrast visual acuity, visualizing missing information, information processing speed (Useful Field of View), visual search, and working memory. Participants were also given a hazard perception test, including 26 silent driving scenes, and 17 scenes that contained a traffic conflict that necessitated an evasive action to avoid a collision with another vehicle, and scenes that did not contain traffic conflict. The on-road driving assessment included parking, intersections, car controls, lane control, traffic lights, speed, right of way, and automatic disqualifications. If a driver exceeded 75 points, they failed the assessment. Some of the mistakes were considered automatic failure such as errors that included right of way violations or a serious safety error.

The Roadwise Review test alone was not proven to predict on-road performance of safety. Of the two, the hazard-perception tests were more accurate in predicting behind-the-wheel outcomes. This test measures adequate physical abilities, visual spatial abilities, cognitive and perceptual systems that support the motor responses needed, working memory, and concentration ability to make the right decisions while driving. This proves that the behind-the-wheel driving assessment, including written and motor testing, will provide the opportunity for the evaluator to most accurately assess the driver's observation skills, judgment, and ability to respond safely to various scenarios while driving. This helps the evaluator to better predict the driver's ability to continue driving, or the need to retire from driving.

Since the individual is impaired early in the progression of dementia to self-regulate, asking the driver if they are safe to drive is likely to be a poor indication of their actual ability to drive safely. Family reports of a person's impaired driving are extremely valuable, but they may not be given enough attention. I spoke with a woman whose husband had caused three accidents- she stated that she reported him to the Department of Motor Vehicles on multiple occasions and asked them to take away his driver's license after the first and second accidents. But the driver's license was only revoked after the third accident, when he caused the death of the other driver. He was leaving a parking lot and made a left turn in front of oncoming traffic (that is the most common cause of an accident for an individual living with dementia). She asked him later at home if he knew that he was in an accident, if he felt anything. He stated that he felt a "bump" and looked at the hood to see if there was any damage, didn't see any, so he kept driving. The only reason he stopped driving was because the front left tire fell off his car. The other car had overturned, but he never saw it rolling over.

Chapter 15

Is Your Loved One Safe To Drive?

Can We Identify the Greatest Risk?

The best predictors of driving impairment with a diagnosis of dementia are disease time span and severity of the symptoms. In a study by Drachman and collaborators, they determined that the risk began to rise significantly after the third year of the disease. They found the maximum crash rate was similar to rates observed in 16- to 24-year old males. However, the miles driven per individual were not similar, since the older drivers (65%) diagnosed with dementia had decreased the miles they drove, unlike the young males. It is interesting that in this study, half of the drivers stopped driving within three years after diagnosis of dementia. It could be significant for medical professionals and family members to follow this study; driving should be assessed by the 3-year mark, or before if warranted. In another study by Friedland et al, the crash rate increased after three years of progressing symptoms. It is also interesting that this study reported that males with

Alzheimer's disease had higher rates of accidents than females in the study but were not shown to have increased cognitive impairment when given the Mini-Mental Status Examination. This is likely due to males having a higher incidence of driving as they age, and tend to take more risks compared to females, who tend to give up driving more readily than do males.

In a study from England, it was reported that 22% of the persons living with dementia continued to drive more than three years after diagnosis; when the physician gave them an assessment for driving safety, the physician reported these drivers to be impaired.

Each individual living with dementia will have a unique response to the disease and will have unique symptoms. Therefore, it is important for the physician to monitor the progression of the disease and the symptoms to restrict driving, and eventually stop the individual from driving before a crash occurs.

I found that it is best to conduct the driving assessment at the individual's home. They feel more comfortable at home and have complete privacy when completing the written portion of the assessment, as opposed to completing the assessment in a hospital or clinic. They are more familiar with the roads and landmarks near their home, and I want to observe their usual driving habits.

The Hartford car insurance company has a wonderful program that they developed with the American Occupational Therapy Association and MIT AgeLab. They stress the importance of talking to the individual before a diagnosis of MCI or dementia, so the individual has plenty of time to get adjusted to the idea that one day they may have to retire from driving. According to their research, drivers over the age of 70 have an increased risk for being involved in an accident. According to a 2015 study by the Insurance Institute for Highway Safety, there is a slightly increased risk of being injured in an accident after age 70, but the increase is dramatic at age 75 and is even more significant after age 85. In their booklet, "We Need to Talk," they give a step-by-step way to approach an older adult to discuss driving safely, and how to talk about impaired driving.

According to their research, it is usually difficult to talk to an older adult about their driving. It is generally more accepted for the older adult to hear concerns from a family member- either a spouse or adult child they trust. Some older adults trust their doctor to talk about this issue. However, it is important to understand that even a person with MCI, much less a diagnosis of dementia, is likely to dismiss concerns presented to them, no matter who is presenting their concerns.

Another reason it is difficult to talk to older adults about concerns is because the individual typically does not want to hear about errors they are making while driving. If the family or doctor can talk to the individual about their concerns, they are generally more open to hearing concerns of issues that may be causing impairment to their driving skills, rather than from a friend or neighbor.

Behind-The-Wheel Test Vs. Driving Simulator

So far, the gold standard for accurate testing has been the on-road assessment. The challenge of this test is that the driver might be more anxious than usual due to driving a car they are not familiar with and having passengers who are observing the driving patterns. Another challenge during the behind-the-wheel test is the evaluator must let the individual make at least part of a mistake before intervening to avoid any serious consequences, e.g. the driver might attempt a left turn in front of oncoming traffic but the driving instructor won't allow the driver to pull out in front of traffic.

Using a driving simulator in testing older adults with a dementia diagnosis can be nerve-wracking for the individual because they are not familiar with simulated driving. However, the advantage of using a driving simulator is that the evaluator can program certain hazards into the test that they may not have the opportunity to observe during a behind-the-wheel test. In one study there were 13 individuals with a dementia diagnosis who were still driving and were tested with the simulator. Six of the subjects were rated in the poor range, and seven subjects performed in the normal range. The poor range scorers also scored lower on the MMSE and other cognitive tests of visual processing and non-verbal capabilities. The simulator clearly augmented the conclusion that they are unable to drive safely.

How driving can be properly evaluated

All driving assessment programs are listed on the American Occupational Therapy Association- www.aota.org. When you choose an occupational therapy driving assessment program, your loved one can be assessed medically as part of determining their physical ability to drive safely. This provides a more thorough, comprehensive assessment. A qualified occupational therapist will be able to provide assessments such as manual muscle tests and range-of-motion for both upper and lower extremities. In addition, the individual will be assessed for cognitive functional skills, physical function, attention span, useful field of view, reaction time, visual processing skills, motor planning skills, and multi-tasking skills. These tests are not included in state motor vehicle departments, nor are they provided in

the test performed by AAA.

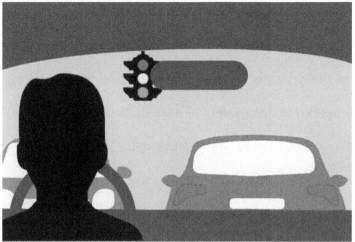

**This Illustrations shows the normal field of view
for a driver with no impairments. In the light blue.**

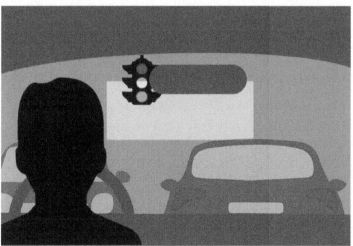

**This illustration demonstrates the area that a
person living with dementia can see and process-
the small box above the first car. A person living
with dementia is no longer able to see everything
that appears in the windshield and respond as
needed. In the light blue.**

The second part of the test is the behind-the-wheel portion when the individual will be observed driving the test car with dual controls for the driving instructor and occupational therapist. This is the hands-on part of the test where the driver will have to demonstrate all the driving skills needed to drive safely. These skills include the ability to follow state driving laws, street signs, and signal lights; ability to stay within the correct lane position; accurate turns; attention span and concentration; memory for way-finding; acceptable response to emergency situations/hazards; leaving adequate space for pedestrians or other vehicles on the road; ability to back the car in a straight line; ability to park accurately; sequencing for starting and parking the car, and general driving skills. The occupational therapist will be observing for the driver's ability to respond appropriately to road hazards, other drivers, whether the individual has inappropriate responses when driving, e.g. road rage, and how they respond when the driving instructor must correct their flawed driving. Every aspect of their driving, from the moment they get in the car to when they exit the car, is observed and is important information to gather for making the final recommendation regarding continued driving or having to retire from driving.

The importance of making the right decision is certainly a big weight on the shoulders of the occupational therapist when making this decision. All the information from the written tests, the observations during the driving test, and the driver's self-assessment has to be put together to make the most appropriate recommendation.

Chapter 16

Legal Consequences of Driving While Living with Dementia

There is precedent being set in California that when an older adult living with dementia causes an accident, the opposing party commonly requests the medical records of the driver. If the medical record contains information about cognitive impairment of any type, that information is submitted with the lawsuit, and these drivers are at risk to lose everything-any assets, their home, a large financial settlement. Your loved one may not understand the implications of this danger, but it is something that you need to consider carefully. If you condone your loved one to continue driving, the loss of assets in a lawsuit tremendously impacts the person's quality of life in the future, especially if they end up needing in-home care or need to move to a facility for 24-hour care, either of which are likely.

If your loved one can no longer drive safely, they will be given the results of the testing, and the reasons for the recommendation by the occupational therapist after the behind-the-wheel test is complete. I report the individual to the state DMV as well, including the critical and non-critical errors, which impact the decision of whether then can or cannot continue to drive.

You can report your loved one to the DMV anonymously in California, but I have heard many stories of DMV employees being "compassionate" and informing the driver of who reported them. That is why I am willing to send in the report- to save the doctor or family the unpleasant confrontation with the driver who is losing their driving privileges.

Chapter 17

Case Studies

Most Common Mistakes that Drivers Living with Dementia Make:

(Disclosure: the age, name, and profession were changed to protect everyone)

The purpose of these case studies is to advise you that cognitive impairment does impact driving and can start in the early stage of impairment, at MCI. These case studies are random examples of educational level completed, different professional histories, scores on the written portion of the test, and the mistakes that were made during the driving portion of the test. There have been hundreds of drivers tested, but I chose to share only ten cases.

CASE STUDY 1:

Ms. Woolen was a 75-year-old woman with a diagnosis of MCI. She was a retired pet groomer; educationally, had completed high school. On the written test she scored 17/30 on the cognitive test, which is in the dementia range. In the motor planning portion of the test, she scored in the severely impaired range. She scored 80% on her knowledge of street signs. On the tests to determine her ability to perform multi-tasking skills, she demonstrated mild impairment on the first four tests, and severe impairment on the last test.

For the on-the-road test, she made multiple rolling stops. This is a common error on the behind-the-wheel portion when testing a person with cognitive impairment. She attempted to make a left turn in front of oncoming traffic, requiring intervention from the driving instructor to avoid an accident. She made wide turns and straddled two lanes at the end of the turns, then merged into another lane. She also did not look over her shoulder prior to making lane changes, which is something that the DMV in California requires when testing drivers. On one portion of the road test, she was driving in a lane that ended, requiring cars to merge left. Her choice was to stop the car when the lane ended and wait until there were no cars in the left lane prior to merging into the lane. When the driving portion of the test was completed and she was instructed to return home, she drove onto the freeway headed in the opposite direction of her home, and once again required intervention from the driving instructor to assist her.

Case Study 2:

Mr. Norton was a 83-year-old male with a diagnosis of stroke who was still working as a consultant for airport safety. He scored 60% on the street signs test, and scored 15/30 on the cognitive function test, which is in the dementia range. On the test for multi-tasking skills, he scored so severely impaired on the first two tests that he was not given the additional three tests. On the driving portion of the test, when he approached an intersection with a green light, he stepped hard on the brakes to stop the car, requiring intervention from the driving instructor to proceed through the intersection. He made 15 rolling stops; he did not stop completely at red lights or stop signs but would step lightly on the brake and continue driving.

Mr. Norton drove on the right side of the lane, in the bike lane, on the Bots dots, and too close to parked cars throughout the assessment. When approaching an intersection where the light had already turned yellow, he continued at full speed and required intervention from the driving instructor to stop the car at the red light. He did not look over his shoulder prior to making lane changes, and twice while attempting a lane change, he required intervention from the driving instructor to avoid hitting a vehicle that occupied the lane. He did not slow down for speed bumps, either on the street or in parking lots. He drove the wrong way down a driveway in a shopping center.

When Mr. Norton was instructed to back out of a parking space safely, he backed the car without looking behind the car, and required intervention to avoid hitting a car that was already backing out of the parking space behind him. When driving through the same parking lot, he did not stop for pedestrians walking in a cross walk, and kept rolling toward them, requiring intervention from the driving instructor.

Another pedestrian had to walk behind the car to avoid getting hit. He drove significantly under the speed limit.

Case Study 3:

Mr. Rasmussen was a 77-year-old male who previously owned an auto parts manufacturing company. He scored mildly impaired on the motor planning test. He scored 17/30 on the cognitive test, which is in the dementia range. He scored mildly impaired on the first multi-tasking test, in the normal range on the second and third tests, mildly impaired on the fourth test, and severely impaired on the fifth test. He stated that he had one recent accident that was not his fault. He recently received a traffic ticket for making a left turn; he stated that there was a new sign stating, "no left turn", and he didn't see the sign.

On the driving portion of the test, Mr. Rasmussen made six short stops- did not complete the stops but rolled through each intersection. At one intersection there were pedestrians in the crosswalk; he kept moving forward on the right turn rather than waiting for the pedestrians to step on the sidewalk as mandated by state law. He attempted to make another right turn in front of oncoming traffic, requiring intervention from the driving instructor to prevent an accident. And at another intersection, he attempted to drive through a crosswalk where pedestrians were entering, again required intervention to avoid hitting the pedestrians.

Case Study 4:

Mr. Rudolph was a 75-year-old who had a career as a car salesman. He scored less than 50% on all four visual processing tests, which tests an individual's ability to see an object in a busy background. He scored severely impaired on the motor planning test and made 6 errors. He scored 12/30 on the cognitive function assessment, which is in the dementia range. When given the multi-tasking test, he scored so severely impaired on the first test that he was not given subsequent tests.

When on the driving test he drove significantly under the speed limit on surface streets. He did not look over his shoulder when making lane changes and required intervention repeatedly to avoid hitting other cars. When stopping at red lights he just kept rolling toward the intersection, again requiring repeated intervention from the driving instructor to stop the car at a safe distance from cars in front. He also rolled through stop signs rather than make a complete stop.

When pedestrians were crossing the street in a crosswalk, he again kept rolling toward the intersection and required intervention from the driving instructor to avoid hitting the pedestrians. When approaching another intersection, he became confused and drove into the left lane, then realized he needed to be in the right lane, and suddenly crossed two lanes to get into the right turn lane. Once he entered the freeway, he started to make a lane change to the left, which was occupied by a large SUV-- the driver of the SUV sped up to avoid a collision.

Mr. Rudolph was driving 75 mph on the freeway, which has a speed limit of 65 mph. When exiting the freeway, he did not turn the steering wheel adequately to stay on the road and was heading toward the curb when the driving instructor grabbed the steering wheel to steer the car back to the exit lane. He also changed lanes in the middle of the exit, without looking to see if the lane was occupied or not. When he entered a parking lot, he continued to drive when pedestrians were walking across the lane, again requiring intervention from the driving instructor to let the pedestrians pass safely.

He was asked to park the car, and then to back up, and when backing he did not observe a car that was already backed up and was close to the test car, once again requiring intervention from the driving instructor to avoid an accident. He was unable to keep the car in the correct lane position, weaving in and out of the lane, and made very wide turns onto the opposite side of the road. When given the results of the testing, and the recommendation that he should retire from driving, he became very angry and started shaking his fists at the test provider.

Case Study 5:

Mr. Taylor was a 76-year-old male who was a reporter for a newspaper. On the motor planning test, he scored severely impaired, and made nine errors. He had a great deal of difficulty taking the road signs test. He scored 8/10 correctly but took over 30 minutes to finish the test. He scored 6/30 on the cognitive function test. When taking the multi-tasking test, he scored so low on the first test that he was not given the remaining four tests.

During the driving test Mr. Taylor did not look over his shoulder prior to making any lane changes. He rolled through stop signs. He did not consistently signal lane changes and turns prior to starting the maneuvers. He drove down the middle of the street, straddling the center line. He forgot the correct sequence for parking the car-- he left the car in Drive, instead of putting the car in Park and turned off the engine, then couldn't figure out why the car wouldn't start when he wanted to leave. He did not follow speed limit signs; for most of the test he drove as much as 20 mph under the speed limit, but at one point he was driving 10 mph over the speed limit. He started a left turn before one intersection and crossed the middle line of the road twice- with both lanes. He started a right turn in the right turn lane, then crossed over the middle line of the turn lanes and straddled the two lanes for the rest of the turn. He had difficulty keeping the car in the correct lane position and drove repeatedly on the Bots dots rather than in the middle of the lane.

When attempting to make a left turn into an alley he started the turn without looking to the right to determine if it was safe to complete the turn. At the next intersection he attempted to make a right turn when two pedestrians were crossing the street, from opposite directions, causing the driving instructor to intervene. When attempting to make a left turn, he missed the turn lane and attempted to cross two lanes from the right lane, again requiring intervention to avoid hitting other cars.

Case Study 6:

Mrs. Pettit was a 92-year-old female who is a retired administrative assistant for the president of a local audio-visual company. On the motor planning test, she scored in the moderately impaired range. She scored 14/30 on the cognitive function test, which is in the dementia range. She scored mildly impaired on the first four multi-tasking tests, then scored severely impaired on the fifth test.

On the driving test Mrs. Pettit did not look over her shoulder prior to making lane changes. She drove very impulsively, making sudden, frequent lane changes. She made rolling stops rather than complete stops at stop signs. Before the driving instructor could intervene, she made a left turn in front of oncoming traffic. When driving through a parking lot she refused to stop for a pedestrian--she kept driving toward the pedestrian. She also stopped too close to cars that were stopped at red lights and did not change this habit even when instructed that she needed to leave adequate space between her car and the car in front. She did not follow speed limit signs and drove 5-10 mph under the speed limit as well as over the speed limit. When stopped at a red light she did not observe when the light turned green and she did not proceed until instructed to move. When parked at a shopping center she forgot how to put the car in the correct gear and required instruction again for the sequencing of changing to the correct gear.

Case Study 7:

Mr. Daniels is a 79-year-old retired professor of anthropology and had a diagnosis of cerebral vascular accident and transient ischemic attack. He scored 22/30 on the cognitive test, which is in the mild neurocognitive impairment range. He scored so severely impaired on the first test of multi-tasking skills that he was not given the subsequent tests. On the motor planning test, he scored in the severely impaired range, with 15 errors.

When driving, Mr. Daniels repeatedly stopped too close to other cars at red lights. Although he was given repeated instruction to stop at a safe distance behind other cars he did not do so. He did not follow speed limit signs, driving up to 30 mph under the speed limit, and 10 mph over the speed limit. He did not look over his shoulder prior to making lane changes and twice required intervention to avoid hitting large trucks that occupied the adjacent lane.

He repeatedly drifted across lanes, drove on the left or right side of the lane, and drove on the Bots dots for extended periods of time. He attempted several turns, and rather than pull over to wait for a safe turn he stopped in the middle of the lane, blocking traffic. At one intersection he was facing a green light, and a pedestrian had a red light, but he stopped and signaled the pedestrian to proceed. He was instructed that he had the right-of-way, and to proceed while he was facing a green light.

In a parking lot Mr. Daniels spotted two pedestrians, but rather than stop for them he continued to drive until the driving instructor intervened to allow the pedestrians to pass safely. He attempted to make a left turn in front of oncoming traffic, requiring intervention to stop until it was safe to turn. At several points during the driving assessment he started crying, saying that he knew he was making mistakes.

Case Study 8:

Mrs. Lowry is 95-year-old retired housewife and she had a diagnosis of dementia. She scored severely impaired on the reaction time test. In testing her multi-tasking skills she scored severely impaired on the first three tests, so was not given the last two tests. She scored moderately impaired on the motor planning test and 17/30 on the cognitive function test, which is in the dementia range. When she was given instruction for how to use the car and was shown where the gas and brake pedals were located, she became very upset because she kept stepping on the gas pedal when she was asked to step on the brake. She was instructed on how to release the parking brake several times, and again became upset, stating that she never uses the parking brake, so she didn't know how to release the brake. She required physical intervention to release the brake.

She did not look over her shoulder prior to making lane changes, even when given repeated instructions to check the lane first. She made abrupt starts and stops and pumped the brake rather than making a smooth stop. She did not slow down for speed bumps on the roads near her home even though she lived on that street for 30 years.

When parking the car in a parking lot, she forgot to shut off the engine after she was asked to go through the correct sequencing of parking. She attempted to back the car out of the parking space and stated she didn't know why the car wasn't moving- she required verbal cues to put the car in reverse prior to leaving the parking space. She drove 10-15 mph over the speed limit. She weaved in and out of the lane, and made multiple rolling stops, rather than complete stops. At one point she turned into a driveway that had a yellow line at the entrance of the driveway. She became very confused and stated that she didn't know what to do next, so was instructed on how to exit the driveway. When she was instructed to park the car next to the curb, she attempted but was not able to back the car in a straight line and ran into the curb. When she attempted to pull away from the curb, she had not changed the gear from reverse, and was surprised that she was backing up. She then stepped on the brake pedal, when attempting to move the car forward, thinking that her foot was on the gas pedal instead of the brake.

Case Study 9:

Mrs. Sumpter is an 82-year-old retired real estate broker. She had diagnoses of Memory Loss, Cataracts, and Heart Arrythmia. She scored in the severely impaired range on the reaction time test. She scored in the normal range on the first multi-tasking skills test, mildly impaired on the next two tests, moderately impaired on the fourth test, and severely impaired on the fifth test. She scored 19/30 on the cognitive function test, which is in the dementia range.

On the driving portion of the test, Mrs. Sumpter's first mistake occurred when she was in a left turn lane and attempted to drive straight through the intersection, requiring intervention from the driving instructor. On the next turn, she attempted to make a left turn in front of oncoming traffic, again requiring intervention from the driving instructor. She did not look over her shoulder prior to making lane changes and required intervention several times to avoid hitting cars that occupied the lanes.

When she approached an intersection with a sign that read "Right Turn Only", she argued with the driving instructor that she should be allowed to make the left turn and became very upset that the driving instructor would not allow her to. She approached a second intersection with a "No U Turn" sign and announced that she was going to make a U-turn. The driving instructor pointed to the sign and stated that she was not legally allowed to make a U-turn there. She then looked at the sign, admitted that the sign said, "No U-Turn," then stated that she was confused and did not know how to continue driving. She stated that she and "many others" regularly made U-turns at that intersection, and "they didn't get tickets", as if to justify her decision. She required intervention to help her proceed through the intersection legally and return home. When leaving that area, she suddenly made a right turn without signaling or braking, causing the car behind us to slam on their brakes to avoid hitting us.

Case Study 10:

Mrs. Ricketts is an 85-year-old female with a diagnosis of Concussion. She scored in the normal range on the first multi-tasking test, scored mildly impaired on the next two, moderately impaired on the fourth test, and severely impaired on the fifth test. She scored mildly impaired on the motor planning test, 40% on the street signs test, and 17/30 on the cognitive function test, which is in the Dementia range.

After being given a thorough orientation to the test car, Mrs. Ricketts stated she was ready to drive. She attempted to pull away from the curb but put the gear in reverse and backed up instead. However, when asked, she was then able to check the gear panel and correctly stated that the car was in reverse. She was able to safety put the car in drive and pull away from the curb.

When driving on the street she attempted to make numerous unsafe lane changes, and twice required intervention because the lanes were occupied by other vehicles. She drove on the wrong side of the road twice, even when driving in her own neighborhood. She drove 15-30 mph under the speed limit throughout the assessment. She was instructed to make a right turn at an intersection, but she stopped at two different locations of the block prior to reaching the intersection.

Conclusion- you can see that there are many similarities with these case studies, with a few individual mistakes. They all had difficulty with multi-tasking skills, poor planning skills, difficulty with keeping the car in the correct lane position. They often break the law by driving through stop signs and red lights, and stop at green lights, but they always justify why they did not follow the law. One male driver, when asked why he didn't stop fully at stop signs, stated that it was "inconvenient" to stop. The typical responses, when given the results of the tests and the recommendation to retire from driving, is that they didn't make the mistakes listed or they were "safe to drive" in spite of the test results, and the "proof" was that "no accident occurred during the driving assessment". It is rare than an individual living with dementia will admit to making driving mistakes. You can see that the age of the drivers in these case studies did not make a significant impact on their driving- it was the cognitive impairment that most affected the driving.

Chapter 18

Statistics and Research

There are over 5.8 million Americans living with dementia and it is estimated that 30-40% still drive. That means that 1,740,000 to 2,320,000 individuals are driving with dementia in the United States. We understand that older adults want to drive- they like the independence to go where they want to go, when they want to go, the ability to live in their own home, maintain a lifestyle they've likely had for decades, and to maintain their identity and sense of self. After all, we are the nation that guarantees freedom and independence, right? They may need the independence of driving due to lack of assistance or believe that they don't have adequate assistance to run errands. The problem is that the people who are driving with dementia often have no clue that they are unsafe to drive, and do not typically retire from driving without intervention from family or medical professionals.

The other major problem that we face is that an individual with cognitive impairment, whether MCI (Mild Cognitive Impairment) or dementia, can have impaired driving even in early stages. If their cognitive impairment progresses, it is guaranteed they will have impaired driving by the time they reach moderate stage dementia. But it is not common knowledge to doctors and other medical professionals, or to the public, that allowing a person with cognitive impairment to drive may be a risk for not only the driver, but all pedestrians and other drivers near the impaired driver.

We know that all drivers with dementia will become too impaired to drive, but it is possible for some people with early stage cognitive impairment to continue driving and may never become an unsafe driver. It is impossible to predict when the person will become so impaired that they are no longer safe to drive. So how do we make that determination?

According to one study by the Center for Disease Control, drivers over the age of 75 have the highest collision rates of any age category and have higher crash death rates. If you add cognitive impairment or any type of dementia such as Alzheimer's disease, the risk of collision increases 2.5 to 4.7 times more when compared to healthy, age-matched individuals. Even drivers with mild dementia have demonstrated increased risk of reduced safety awareness during an on-road driving assessment. Among other problems, a common mistake I have seen on the driving portion of the test is that drivers with dementia often fail to demonstrate an appropriate response to hazards on the road, increasing risk of causing an accident.

There has been an ongoing debate among medical professionals as to how the driving performance should be evaluated. What is the most accurate way to assess whether a driver with cognitive impairment is safe or unsafe to drive? Each state has a motor vehicle department that uses a number system to determine if unsafe driving behaviors are present. This approach does not delineate the difference between common driving errors and more hazardous errors that might indicate a significant decline in driving safety, so an on-road performance assessment was created for healthy older adults, focusing on these three areas: hazardous infractions, total points accumulated, and comprehensive pass-fail assessments.

In a study by Jones Ross RW, et al in 2014, they used The Roadwise Review from AAA, and the hazard perception test, along with other vision tests to determine which combination of tests had the most predictive validity.

During the first of two sessions they tested participants for visual ability and visual processing skills. In the second session they used the MMSE (Mini Mental Status Exam) and the Roadwise Review. The Roadwise Review has eight subtests: leg strength and general mobility, head and neck flexibility, high-contrast visual acuity, low-contrast visual acuity, visualizing missing information, information processing speed, visual search, and working memory. Participants were also given a hazard perception test, including scenes that contained a traffic conflict that necessitated an evasive action to avoid a collision with another vehicle. The last scenes did not contain a traffic conflict.

The on-road driving assessment included parking, intersections, car controls, lane control, traffic lights, speed, right of way, and automatic disqualifications.

The Roadwise Review test alone was not proven to predict on-road performance of safety. Of the two, the hazard perception tests were more accurate in predicting behind-the-wheel outcomes. This test measures adequate physical abilities, visual spatial abilities, cognitive and perceptual systems that support the motor responses needed, working memory, and the ability to concentrate to make the right decisions while driving. This proves that the behind-the-wheel driving assessment, including written and motor testing, will provide the opportunity for the evaluator to most accurately assess the driver's observation skills, judgment, and ability to respond safely to various scenarios while driving. This enables the evaluator to better predict the driver's ability to continue driving, or the need to retire from driving.

Sex of Individual - Pertaining to Driving

Studies show with drivers 70 and older that there is an increased likelihood of an accident being caused by males as opposed to females. One explanation is that males often take increased risks when driving. Studies have determined that older women tend to stop driving earlier in the cognitive impairment disease process than men, thereby giving older men greater opportunities for causing an accident than an older female.

Some clients will admit that they have concerns about their own driving and will accept the recommendation to retire from driving. But it is typically the men who have the most protests for driving cessation. When a male client is informed that he is no longer safe to drive, the response heard most often is, "I will die if I can't drive". Female clients who are instructed to stop driving have run the gamut of being accepting of the recommendation to stop driving, but some have also protested and stated that the testing was not valid. Or they try to negotiate, saying that they will only drive to the grocery store or other destinations close to home. If an individual living with dementia is deemed unsafe to drive, it means they are unsafe to drive to any destination. **This means no destination is safe, whether it is one mile or twenty.**

Chapter 19

Alternative Transportation

If an individual is no longer safe to drive, it is important that they are given alternatives. There are some driving alternatives in Southern California that may not be an option for you, so you need to research what is available in your area.

This will vary according to where you live, so you may not have some of the resources that are listed:

- Taxis- call your local senior center and inquire about discounted taxi vouchers
- Local Senior Centers- may have free or low-cost car and/or van rides. At the senior center in Huntington Beach there are 500 volunteer drivers who will drive a senior citizen door to door within city limits. This senior center also has a bus that will take their members anywhere within city limits as well as to the large hospital nearby: the cost is $3.95 per ride.

- GoGo Grandparent- they contract with Uber to hire drivers who have been trained as caregivers and will drive the person door to door and assist with walkers or wheelchairs if needed. They will not stay with the individual, so this is not a viable option for someone needing assistance after they reach the destination. Contact information is gogograndparent.com

- Local home care agencies- some provide a trained caregiver and rides to appointments, shopping, etc. The caregiver will stay with the individual and will assist them throughout the trip, unlike gogograndparent.com, which only provides rides. An example of a national caregiver agency providing rides and will stay with the individual is Right At Home (877-697-7537).

- Friends and/or family

- Private driver- Individuals with the financial ability can hire a private driver or limo service. Be very careful about hiring an individual for driving. You must do a background check, check driving records, employment records, and get multiple references.

- Uber/Lyft- the problem with this option is that many older adults don't have a smart phone, or if they do, they don't know how to use the feature of requesting these rides. Your option is to contact these services FOR your loved one.

- Subway- may be a viable option in beginning stages of dementia only. The individual needs to be tested to determine their safety with riding mass transit options.

- City buses- may be a viable option unless learning something new provides challenges to the individual. May be too complicated to use after a dementia diagnosis.

WARNING: I do not recommend trying to teach someone living with dementia how to use a mass transit system if they have never used one before. It is unlikely that the individual will be able to follow through with the instructions and will probably not be able to use the system accurately. Even if the individual has experience riding on mass transit, it does not mean they will continue to have the ability after a diagnosis of dementia. It is likely for them to make mistakes such as getting on the wrong train or getting off at the wrong exit. There is no consistency guaranteed with learned skills after a diagnosis of cognitive impairment.

Chapter 20

In Conclusion

As of this writing I started my driving assessment company 19 years ago. Prior to starting my company, I had a private practice where I was providing cognitive stimulation exercises to clients who had a diagnosis of dementia. I started observing that some of these clients were still driving. One client of mine was involved in four accidents. I asked her husband why he let her continue to drive. He stated that she would be "really upset" if he forced her to stop driving. Rather than doing the hard thing he bought an umbrella insurance policy to cover her in case of future accidents.

I then realized these clients needed a driving assessment, since they demonstrated significant memory loss during my therapy sessions with them. I took classes to learn how to provide driving assessments. Then hired a driving instructor with a dual control vehicle to work with me so that I could also provide a **safe** behind-the-wheel assessment. I found that I was not passing driver after driver causing me to wonder if I was being too harsh with my evaluations. Was there was validity to my testing conclusions that there were so many unsafe drivers on the road? I spoke with a friend, the Manager of a Driver Safety Office of the DMV, and spoke with him about the number of drivers not passing the driving test. He assured me that there were, indeed, many unsafe drivers on the road who continue to drive. Not all unsafe drivers were being reported to the DMV for their driving. I also spoke with my friend and business partner, Dr. Kent Peppard (PhD), a neuropsychologist as well as one of the nation's leading experts on testing individuals with cognitive impairment. He has given to me the most consistent support and encouragement to continue testing these individuals. Thus, helping me to realize that I am providing a community service by helping unsafe drivers to stop driving, and probably saving lives.

I had a very disturbing case where the gentleman I tested made many serious errors. When I was giving him feedback on his test results, I recommended that he had to stop driving. He became very upset; more than any other individual I have tested to this day. He told me repeatedly that he would die if he couldn't drive, that he needed food, supplies, and the freedom to do what he wanted. After two hours of talking to him, he stated that he was going to kill himself. I asked him if he had a plan, and he stated that he owned two guns and planned to put bullets in the guns, put the guns to his head, and kill himself. I realized at that point I might be in danger, and I left. I called Dr. Peppard about the situation, and he advised me to contact authorities, so I did. He also reassured me, again, that the work I am doing is saving lives, and that the community needs this service.

I found that many family members openly expressed that they were grateful to me for informing their loved one they were no longer safe to drive. Many physicians have also expressed gratitude that they were able to maintain the professional relationship with their patient as they did not have to become involved in the process of taking away driving privileges.

The biggest challenge for you will be persuading your patient or loved one to be tested for driving safety. It is not an easy journey for all individuals involved, but it is better that the driver is tested and prevented from making a serious driving error, resulting in harm to themselves or others. We need to support older adults to drive, as long as they remain safe to drive, and find alternate transportation for those who are no longer safe to drive.

Bibliography

Alzheimer's Association. Giving up the car keys. *National Newsletter.* 1995; 3:1, 7
Post SG, Whitehouse P. Fairhill guidelines of the care of people with Alzheimer's
disease: a clinical summary. *J Am Geriatr Soc.* 1995; 43:1423–1429
Mace NL, Rabins PV. The 36-Hour Day. Baltimore, Md: *Johns Hopkins
University Press*; 1991.

American Psychiatric Association *Diagnostic and Statistical Manual of Mental
Disorders DSM-IV-TR Fourth Edition (Text Revision)* American Psychiatric
Publishing; 4ᵗʰ edition 2000.

Agronin, Marc E. *Alzheimer Disease and Other Dementias* (2ⁿᵈ Edition), Lippincott
Williams & Wilkins, USA, 2008.

Barclay LL, Weiss EM, Mattis S, Bond O, Blass JP. Unrecognized cognitive
impairment in cardiac rehabilitation patients. *J Am Geriatr Soc.* 1988
Jan;36(1):22-8.

Brod M, Schmitt E, Goodwin M, Hodgkins P, Niebler G. ADHD burden of illness
in older adults: a life course perspective. *Qual Life Res.* 2012 Jun;21(5):795-9.

Brown LB, Stern RA, Cahn-Weiner DA, et al. Driving Scenes sub-test of the
Neuropsychological Assessment Battery and on-road driving performance in
aging and very mild dementia. *Arch Clin Neuropsychol.* In press

Budson, A.E. & Soloman, P.R. *Memory Loss: A Practical Guide for Clinicians*
Elsevier Health Sciences 2011.

Budson AE, Solomon PR. New criteria for Alzheimer disease and mild cognitive
impairment: implications for the practicing clinician.
Neurologist. 2012 Nov;18(6):356-63.

Campbell MK, Bush TL. Medical conditions associated with driving cessation in
community- dwelling ambulatory drivers. J Gerontol. 1993;48:S230–S234.

Carr D, Jackson T, Alguire P. Characteristics of an elderly driving population
referred to a geriatric assessment center. J Am Geriatr Soc. 1990;38:1145–1150.

Caycedo AM, Miller B, Kramer J, Rascovsky K. Early features in frontotemporal
dementia. *Curr Alzheimer Res.* 2009 Aug;6(4):337-40.

Center for Disease Control and Prevention
Federal Highway Administration, US Department of Transportation, Highway
Statistics, 2009, Washington, DC.

Cooper PJ, Tallman K, Tuokko H, Beattie BL. Vehicle crash involvement and
cognitive deficit in older drivers. *J Safety Res.* 1993;24:9-17.

Cotrell V, Wild K. Longitudinal study of self-imposed driving restrictions and
deficits awareness in patients with Alzheimer disease. *Alzheimer Dis Assoc
Disord.* 1999; 13:151–156.

Cox DJ, Quillian WC, Thorndike FP. Evaluating driving performance of
outpatients with Alzheimer disease. J Am Board Fam Pract. 1998;11:264–271.

Croisile B, Auriacombe S, Etcharry-Bouyx F, Vercelletto M; National Institute on Aging (u.s.); Alzheimer Association. [The new 2011 recommendations of the National Institute on Aging and the Alzheimer's Association on diagnostic guidelines for Alzheimer's disease: Preclinal stages, mild cognitive impairment, and dementia]. Rev Neurol (Paris). 2012 Jun;168(6-7):471-82. [Article in French]

Crum, R.M., Anthony, J.C., Bassett, S. S., & Folstein, M.F. (1993) Population-based norms for the Mini-mental State Examination by age and education level, *JAMA* 269, 2386-2391.

Cummings JL, Dubois B, Molinuevo JL, Scheltens P. International Work Group criteria for the diagnosis of Alzheimer disease. *Med Clin North Am.* 2013 May;97(3):363-8.

Dash, P. & Villemarette-Pittman, N. (2005) *Alzheimer's Disease*. AAN

Dobbs, B.M., Carr, D.B., & Morris, J.C. (2002). Evaluation and management of the driver with dementia. *The Neurologist,* Vol. 8/No.2.

Dobbs AR, Heller RB, Schopflocher D. A comparative approach to identifying unsafe older drivers. *Accid Anal Prev* 1998;30:363-370.

Drachman DA, Swearer JM the Collaborative Group. Driving and Alzheimer's disease: the risk of crashes. *Neurology.* 1993;43:2448–2456.

Dubinsky RM, Williamson A, Gray CS, et al. Driving in Alzheimer's disease. *J Am Geriatr Soc* 1992;40:1112-1116

Duchek JM, Carr DB, Hunt L et al. Longitudinal driving performance in early-stage dementia of the Alzheimer's type. *J Am Geriatr Soc* 2003;51:1342-1347.

Duchek JM, Hunt L, Ball K, et al. Attention and driving performance in Alzheimer's disease. *J Gerontol B Psychol Sci Soc Sci.* 1998;53:P130–141

Evan L., Traffic Safety, Bloomfield Hills, MI, *Science Serving Society*, 2004.

Farnsworth D. Farnsworth 100 Hue and Dichotomous tests for color vision. *J Opt Soc Am* 1943;33:568-578

Fischer BL, Gunter-Hunt G, Steinhafel CH, Howell T. The identification and assessment of late-life ADHD in memory clinics. *J Atten Disord.* 2012 May;16(4):333-8.

Foley DJ, Masaki KH, Ross GW, White LR. *Journal of the American Geriatrics Society.* 2000 August. 48(8). 928-30.

Folstein, M.F., Folstein, S.E. & McHugh, P.R. (1975) Mini-Mental State: A practical method for grading the cognitive state of patients for the clinician. *Journal of Psychiatric Research,* 12, 189-198.

Freedman, M., et al. *Clock Drawing: A Neuropsychological Analysis.* Oxford University Press. 1994.

Friedland RP, Loss E, Kumar A, et al. Motor vehicle crashes in dementia of the Alzheimer type. *Ann Neurol.* 1988;24:782-786.

Gallo, Joseph J., Reichel, William & Anderson, Lillian M. *Handbook of Geriatric Assessment, 2nd Edition* Aspen Publishers, Inc., Gaithersburg, Maryland 1995.

Gilley DW, Wilson RS, Bennett DA, et al. Cessation of driving and unsafe motor vehicle operation by dementia patients. *Arch Intern Med.* 1991;151:941–946.

Golomb J, Kluger A, Ferris SH. Mild cognitive impairment: historical development and summary of research. *Dialogues Clin Neurosci.* 2004 Dec;6(4):351-67.

Grace J, Amick MM, D'abreu A, et al. Neuropscyhological deficits associated with driving performance in Parkinson's and Alzheimer's disease. *J Int Neuropsychol Soc* 2005; 11:766-775.

Grundman, M., et al. Mild cognitive impairment can be distinguished from Alzheimer disease and normal aging for clinical trials. *Arch Neurol.* 2004 Jan;61(1): 11-27

Hodges JR. Alzheimer's disease and the frontotemporal dementias: contributions to clinico-pathological studies, diagnosis, and cognitive neuroscience. *J Alzheimers Dis.* 2013;33 Suppl 1:S211-7.

Hunt LA, Morris JC, Edwards D, Wilson BS. Driving performance in persons with mild senile
dementia of the Alzheimer type. J Am Geriatr Soc. 1993;41:747–753.
Harvey R, Fraser D, Bonner D, et al. Dementia and driving: results of a semi-realistic simulator study. *Int J Geriatr Psychiatry.* 1995;10:859–864

Hunt LA, Murphy CF, Carr D, et al. Reliability of the Washington University Road Test. Arch Neurol. 1997;54:707–712.

Ivanchak N, Fletcher K, Jicha GA. Attention-deficit/hyperactivity disorder in older adults: prevalence and possible connections to mild cognitive impairment. *Curr Psychiatry Rep.* 2012 Oct;14(5):552-60.

Janke MK. Accidents, mileage, and the exaggeration of risk. Accid Anal Prev. 1991;23:183–188.

Kral, VA. Senescent forgetfulness: benign and malignant. *Can Med Assoc J.* 1962 Feb 10;86:257-60.

Kuhn, Daniel *Alzheimer's Early Stages: First Steps for Families, Friends, and Caregivers*
2nd Edition, Hunter House Publishers, Alameda, CA 2003.

Logsdon RG, Teri L, Larson EB. Driving and Alzheimer's disease. J Gen Intern Med.
1992;7:583–588

Loring, D.W. (Editor) *INS Dictionary of Neuropsychology and Clinical Neurosciences,*
2nd Edition, Oxford University Press, New York 2015.

Lucas-Blaustein MJ, Filipp L, Dungan C, Tune L. Driving in patients with dementia. *J Am Geriatr Soc.* 1988;36:1087-1091

McKeith IG, Galasko D, Kosaka K et al. Consensus guidelines for the clinical and pathological diagnosis of dementia with Lewy bodies (DLB): report of the consortium on DBL international workshop. *Neurology* 1996: 47:1113-1124.

O'Neill D, Neubauer K, Boyle M, et al. Dementia and driving. J R Soc Med. 1992;85:199–202

Ott BR, Lafleche G, Whelihan WM, et al. Impaired awareness of deficits in Alzheimer disease. *Alzheimer Dis Assoc Disorders*. 1996; 10:68–76.

Owlsley C, Sloane ME, Ball K et al. Visual-cognitive-correlates of vehicle collisions in older drivers. Psychol Aging 1991;6403-415.

Palmqvist S, Hertze J, Minthon L, Wattmo C, Zetterberg H, Blennow K, Londos E, Hansson O.
Comparison of brief cognitive tests and CSF biomarkers in predicting Alzheimer's disease in mild cognitive impairment: six-year follow-up study. *PLoS One*. 2012;7(6):e38639.

Perry, R., McKeith, I., Perry, E. (Editors) *Dementia with Lewy Bodies Clinical, Pathological, and Treatment Issues* Cambridge University Press, United Kingdom, 1996.

Petersen, Ronald C. (Ed) *Mild Cognitive Impairment: Aging to Alzheimer's Disease*
Oxford University Press, USA, 2003.

Petersen RC. Mild cognitive impairment as a diagnostic entity. J Intern Med. 2004-Sep;256(3): 183-94.

Petersen, R.C., Smith, G.E., Waring, S.C., Ivnik, R.J. Tangalos, E.G., Kokmen, E. Mild cognitive impairment: clinical characterization and outcome. *Arch Neurol*. 1999 Mar;56(3):303-8.

Peterson R, Negash S. *CNS Spectr*. Vol 13, No 1. 2008
Preusser D, Williams A, Ferguson S et al. Fatal crash risk for older drivers at intersections, *Accid Anal Prev* 1998;30151-159.

Peterson, Ronald C. (Ed) *Mild Cognitive Impairment: Aging to Alzheimer's Disease*
Oxford University Press, USA, 2003.

Phillips LA. Delirium in geriatric patients: identification and prevention. *Medsurg Nurs*. 2013 Jan-Feb;22(1):9-12.

Rebok GW, Keyl PM, Bylsma FW, et al. The effects of Alzheimer's disease on driving-related abilities. Alzheimer Dis Assoc Disord. 1994;4:228–240.

Reisberg B, Ferris SH, Kluger A, Franssen E, Wegiel J, de Leon MJ. Mild cognitive impairment (MCI): a historical perspective. *Int Psychogeriatr*. 2008 Feb;20(1):18-31.

Rizzo M, McGehee DV, Dawson JD, Andersen JN. Simulated car crashes at intersections in drivers with Alzheimer's disease. Alzheimer Dis Assoc Disord. 2001;15:10–20.

Roger MA, Welsh RW, Watson S et.al. The relationship between neuropsychological functioning and driving ability in dementia: A meta-analysis. *Neuropsychology* 2004;18:85-93.

Rönnemaa E, Zethelius B, Lannfelt L, Kilander L. Vascular risk factors and dementia: 40-year follow-up of a population-based cohort. *Dement Geriatr Cogn Disord*. 2011;31(6):460-6.

Scialfa CT, Adams E, Giovanetto M. Reliability of the Vistech Contrast Test System in a life-span sample. Optum Vis Sci 1991;30:363-370.

Scialfa CT, Ference J, Boone J, et al. Predicting older adults' driving difficulties using the Roadwise Review. *J Gerenot B Psychol Sci Soc Sci* 2010;65B:434-437.

Schuurmans MJ, Deschamps PI, Markham SW, et al. The measurement of delirium: review of rating scales. *Res Theory Nurs Pract* 2003; 17(3):207-224.

Snowdon, D. *Aging with Grace: The Nun Study* Bantam Books New York 2002.

Storandt, Martha & VandenBos, Gary R. (Eds) *Neuropsychological Assessment of Dementia and Depression in Older Adults: A Clinician's Guide* American Psychological Association, Washington DC 1997.

Strub, R. L. & Black, F. W. *The Mental Status Examination in Neurology.* F. A. Davis Company 2000.

Stutts J, Martell C, Staplin L, Identifying behaviors and situations associated with increased crash risk for older drivers. National Highway Traffic Safety Administration 2009. Report DOT HS 811 093.

Taipa R, Pinho J, Melo-Pires M. Clinico-pathological correlations of the most common neurodegenerative dementias. *Front Neurol.* 2012;3:68.

Tang H, Mao X, Xie L, Greenberg DA, Jin K. Expression level of vascular endothelial growth factor in hippocampus is associated with cognitive impairment in patients with Alzheimer's disease. *Neurobiol Aging.* 2013 May;34(5):1412-5

Tariot PN. Early diagnosis and management of Alzheimer's disease. *J Clin Psychiatry.* 2013 May;74(5):e10.

The Lund Manchester Groups. Clinical and neuropathological criteria for Frontotemporal dementia. *Journal of Neurology, Neurosurgery and Psychiatry* 1994; 57:416-418.

Trzepacz P, Baker R, Greenhouse J. A symptom rating scale for delirium. *Psychiatry Res* 1988;23:89-97.

Tuokko H, Tallman K, Beattie BL, et al. An examination of driving records in a dementia clinic. *J Gerontol B Psychol Sci Soc Sci.* 1995;50B:S173-S181.

Types of dementia. Alzheimer's Society UK   2013.

Tuokko H, Beattie BL, Tallman K, Cooper P. Predictors of motor vehicle crashes in a dementia clinic population: the role of gender and arthritis. J Am Geriatr Soc. 1995;43:1444–1445.

U.S. Dept of Health and Human Services *Recognition and initial assessment of Alzheimer's disease and related dementias* (SuDoc HE 20.6520:19)

U.S. Dept. of Health and Human Services, Public Health Service, Agency for Health Care Policy and Research 1996.

Van der Mussele S, Le Bastard N, Vermeiren Y, Saerens J, Somers N, Mariën P, Goeman J, De Deyn PP, Engelborghs S. Behavioral symptoms in mild cognitive impairment as compared with Alzheimer's disease and healthy older adults. *Int J Geriatr Psychiatry.* 2012 Apr 30.

Vascular Dementia Alzheimer's Association http://www.alz.org/dementia/vascular-dementia-symptoms.asp

Wijeratne C. Behaviour and biomarkers in frontotemporal dementia: implications for general psychiatry. *Aust N Z J Psychiatry.* 2012 May;46(5):477-9.

Wild K, Cotrell V. Identifying driving impairment in Alzheimer disease: a comparison of self and observer reports versus driving evaluation. *Alzheimer Dis Assoc Disord.* 2003; 17:27–34

Made in the USA
Coppell, TX
16 December 2022

89710841R00089